D0801069

SISTERS
OF THE
SOMME

TRUE STORIES FROM
A FIRST WORLD WAR
FIELD HOSPITAL

PENNY STARNS

The History Press

This book is dedicated to all the brave men and women who served at the Order of St John Ambulance Brigade Hospital between 4 September 1915 and 3 March 1919.

Cover illustrations: front (© Corbis); back, Order of St John Knight of Grace badge (Dave Boven).

First published 2016

The History Press
The Mill, Brimscombe Port
Stroud, Gloucestershire, GL5 2QG
www.thehistorypress.co.uk

© Penny Starns, 2016

The right of Penny Starns to be identified as the Author of this work has been asserted in accordance with the Copyright, Designs and Patents Act 1988.

British Library Cataloguing in Publication Data.
A catalogue record for this book is available from the British Library.

ISBN 978 0 7509 6162 2

Typesetting and origination by The History Press
Printed in Great Britain

CONTENTS

ACKNOWLEDGEMENTS

The process of writing this book has been greatly assisted by the staff of the Order of St John Museum, St John's Gate, Clerkenwell, London. In particular, Tom Foakes, Abigail Turner, Hannah Agass, Charlotte Dickerson and Norman Gooding. Collectively they ensured that I had access to unique and fascinating primary source material contained within the Order of St John archive. They gave me their time and valuable insights into the humanitarian history of the Order, for which I am very grateful.

I extend special thanks to Mrs Eva Witton, great niece of VAD Veronica Nisbet, for giving me intimate details of Veronica's character and lifestyle.

I am indebted to my editor Sophie Bradshaw for her knowledge and guidance. I also thank my father for his constant support and encouragement.

In addition, I am grateful to those who have supported the research process by listening patiently to my ideas. These include Matthew Winstone, Michael and Rocha Brown, Joanna Denman, Catherine Nile, Pauline Hancock and Margaret Taplin.

INTRODUCTION

This book adopts a new approach to First World War history by
providing an intimate account of life in one base field hospital.
It is based on the archive material belonging to the Museum of
the Order of St John and other historical documents associated
with the planning and work of the Order of St John Ambulance
Brigade Hospital between 1914 and 1918. It documents both
the routine and drama of field hospital life in France during the
First World War, and follows the lives and interrelationships of
hospital staff and patients. By focussing on one field hospital, this
book sheds light not only on medical procedures, technologies
and medicines but also on the levels of intimacy that were
shared on a daily basis between people of varying backgrounds.
Archive materials, in the form of diaries, letters, first-aid
manuals, supply order books, military standing orders and
official logbooks, detail everything from the weather, numbers
of casualties, their treatment and medical outcomes, changes
in hospital routine, boundary limits for medical personnel and
patients, shortages of gauze dressings, the soaring price of coke
used to fuel the stoves, burst pipes, blocked drains and some
ongoing difficulties with electrical equipment. In amongst the
mundane, however, records reveal the extraordinary nature
of the Order of St John staff; the calm efficiency with which
casualties were admitted, screened, treated and bedded down;
and the immense bravery of personnel who often went above
and beyond the call of duty in order to deliver urgently needed
medical care to the severely injured.

In terms of archive material, special mention needs to be made of an article written by Lieutenant Colonel Ronnie Cole-Mackintosh entitled 'The St John Ambulance Brigade Hospital in Étaples'. The lieutenant colonel fully intended to write and publish a book about the hospital but unfortunately passed away before he had chance to fulfil this ambition. The article he wrote for the Order of St John Historical Society is fascinating and detailed in its content, and it forms an important legacy.

In addition to the wealth of primary source material held at the Order of St John Museum, further documents held at the National Archive have also been consulted. These include War Office files, General Nursing Council files, treasury files, and Her Majesty's Stationery Office (HMSO) advisory leaflets. A wide variety of documents held at the Royal College of Nursing Archives and the Imperial War Museum also contribute to the overall text of this book. Secondary material has been supplied by H. Cushing, *From a Surgeon's Journal* (1936), M. Baly, *Florence Nightingale and the Nursing legacy* (1986) and the author's published PhD thesis 'March of the Matrons' (2000).

The Order of St John of Jerusalem

In 1099 a group of monks in Jerusalem, under the direction of Brother Gerard, founded a hospital to care for sick pilgrims who were on their way to visit the Holy Land. Known as the hospitallers, those who cared for the sick did so in a way that was influenced directly by their Christian beliefs. All pilgrims, regardless of their race or creed, were cared for equally. Hospitallers were instructed to treat every patient as though they were caring for Christ himself. Therefore drinks were given in silver goblets and food was served to patients on a silver platter. From these humble beginnings of service and devout piousness, the Order of St John of Jerusalem was established, and it received official Church recognition in 1113. Once Jerusalem had been conquered during the Crusades, the hospitallers became the Knights of the Order of St John, and from this point on the Order adopted a military–religious role. The Order later branched out and initiated a number of worldwide humanitarian movements. The St John Ambulance Association in Great Britain was established in 1877, followed by the St John Ambulance Brigade in 1887. There was greater female involvement in the British Brigade during the early part of the twentieth century, and by 1915 women had taken on a variety of men's jobs within the St John Voluntary Aid Detachments. Establishing the Brigade Hospital in Étaples was the Order's most important initiative during the First World War. The Order of St John continues to fund a number of humanitarian projects throughout the world, and its influence remains undiminished.

The Field Hospital

In October 1914 the humanitarian organisation of the Order of St John of Jerusalem approached senior ministers at the British Government War Office and offered to provide a 520-bedded base hospital for the purposes of caring for wounded Allied personnel serving on the front line. This offer was duly accepted by the War Office, and £91,000 was raised by the British public by the end of 1914, in order to fund the building of the hospital.

Constructed in a prefabricated hut style, buildings were shipped across to Northern France and built according to the architect's plan. In this way eighteen wards were established. These were divided into two straight lines, which were connected by a series of covered walkways, either side of an administration block. There were sixteen wards of thirty beds and two wards of twenty beds, eleven surgical and six medical. One of the smaller wards was reserved for the treatment of officers. Plaques above individual patient beds displayed the badge of the Order of St John in black and white, and all blankets were a silver grey with the same black-and-white Order badge placed at the centre. The hospital also boasted a modern laboratory and electro-cardiograph department, along with two operating theatres and an X-ray department.

The Order of St John of Jerusalem Ambulance Brigade Hospital was based at Étaples on the north coast of France and quickly became known simply as the Brigade Hospital. Staff consisted of a commanding officer, seventeen medical officers and surgeons, a dental surgeon, a quartermaster and secretary, a matron, an assistant matron, fifty-three trained nurses, twenty-four Voluntary Aid Detachment nurses (VADs) and 141 orderlies, all from the St John Ambulance Brigade and organised as a provisional company. The hospital was unique in many respects. The establishment was underpinned by a strong Christian ethos and almost entirely funded by voluntary contributions. The staff were trained and appointed by the St John Ambulance Brigade, and there was an efficient and crucial staff exchange scheme in operation between the hospital and the 130th St John field ambulance front-line unit. It was also the only hospital within the British Expeditionary Force to have the use of an electrocardiograph machine. This was the first time the machine had been used on active service. Throughout the war the hospital admitted primarily stretcher cases and 'sitters'; the walking wounded were usually cared for elsewhere. There was an added strain on medical staff therefore, in that the hospital always admitted the most severely injured.

The first casualties admitted by St John's arrived on 7 September 1915 at 11.30 p.m.* These patients were from Loos and consisted of a convoy of fifty-seven stretcher cases; they were bedded down by 1.30 a.m. From then on casualties arrived

---

*   Some historians have stated that the first casualties arrived at St John's on
8 September 1915. This is incorrect, however, since the commanding officer's
logbook, held at the Order of St John Museum, and his official letter to the War
Office clearly states that casualties first arrived on 7 September at 11.30 p.m.
For those who wish to read the official logbooks of St John's commanding
officers and the diaries of other members of medical staff, please consult the
Order of St John Museum, Clerkenwell, London. Please also see the National
Archive War Office records, in particular W.O./95/4114 – a series of weekly
letters written from the Commanding Officer of the Order of St John Brigade
Hospital to the War Office between 1915 and 1918.

in various quantities, and at times the injured were overflowing into the hospital corridors on stretchers, trolleys and makeshift mattresses. By the time the Battle of the Somme commenced, the number of hospital beds had increased to 744, and even this number was not enough to provide adequate care for the endless stream of severely injured men. Sometimes hospital staff were given advanced warning of incoming wounded, but if communication lines were down then casualties would arrive unannounced. In terms of the medical care they received, however, casualties had no cause for complaint. The Brigade staff had an excellent reputation. Indeed, the commanding officer of the hospital during the Battle of the Somme, Colonel Trimble, drew attention to the fact that the Order of St John was able to call upon the services of eminent medical men and also the fact that there were few changes of staff, which ensured stability and continuity of care. During the course of the First World War, St John's admitted and treated 36,100 men.

The Battle of the Somme

The Battle of the Somme began on 1 July 1916 and drew to a close on 13 November the same year. Initially conceived as a major Anglo–French offensive in the region of the River Somme, the strategic operational planning quickly became a predominantly British concern. Earlier in the year, the Germans had bombarded the French fortress at Verdun, and substantial numbers of French troops were still embroiled in this rearguard skirmish. Thus the Commander in Chief of the British Army, General Douglas Haig, along with other members of the British High Command, devised battle plans for the Somme offensive, which remain controversial to the present day.

According to these plans, British troops were to attack a 24km front between Serre and Curlu, which lay north of the Somme, whilst available French troops were to attack a 13km front to the south of the Somme. To prepare for these attacks, the Allies bombarded German lines with over 1.5 million artillery shells during the last week of June. Then, at 7.30 a.m. on 1 July, the battle commenced. Imbued with a misplaced confidence, the British high command ordered eleven British divisions to walk towards the German lines. The Germans, meanwhile, had been entrenched in heavily fortified underground bunkers during the earlier shelling and simply assumed new positions at their machine guns when the shelling stopped.

Therefore, as British troops slowly advanced towards the German lines, German machine guns systematically mowed them down, resulting in the indiscriminate slaughter of thousands. By the end of the day 60 per cent of the officers involved in the battle were fatally wounded. Twenty thousand British soldiers were killed and a further 60,000 injured, and yet despite these severe losses, General Haig remained convinced that further attacks of a similar nature would ultimately achieve an Allied victory. However, whole units had been gunned down, and eventually Haig conceded that perhaps limited advances on the southern sector might be more successful. From mid-July to mid-September a stalemate ensued, and neither Allied nor German troops made much headway.[*] French troops had made some gains initially, but they were unable to consolidate these without British support.

---

[*] For those who wish to gain a more detailed knowledge of Allied progress on the Somme please consult the following records, which are held at the National Archive:

W.O.158/322-326, 327-331: These files contain daily reports on the Battle of the Somme July–November 1916 from the Fourth Army Headquarters.

W.O. 161/79: Summary of operations on the Battle of the Somme compiled by the Fourth Army Headquarters.

C.A.B. 45/166: Historical Branch of the Committee of Imperial Defence contains a translated German war diary detailing German military operations 1916.

W.O. 297/5903-5905: Details official French military action during the Battle of the Somme July 1916.

W.O. 153/153-209: An assortment of trench maps of the area around the Somme 1916.

W.O. 297/5926-5927: An assortment of trench maps detailing Allied advances on the Somme July–November 1916.

On 15 September Haig initiated a further British offensive, but by October inclement weather had turned battlefields into mud baths, and on 13 November the battle was over. Casualty numbers were high. British casualties numbered 420,000 and the French recorded nearly 200,000 injured. The Allies had gained a mere 8km of territory.

British Nursing

On the eve of the First World War, British nursing lacked any clear professional identity and was still grappling with recruitment problems and training issues. For much of the nineteenth century, the sick were cared for by relatives and friends more often than by individuals in possession of recognisable nursing skills. Additional care was provided when necessary by religious sisterhoods and domestic handywomen. Disturbingly, the public image of nursing was, for many years, coloured by Charles Dickens and his 'Mrs Sairy Gamp, a gin soaked domestic woman of ill repute and dubious hygiene standards'. Given this appalling stereotype, it was perhaps not surprising that respectable women had shied away from the idea of embarking on a nursing career. Military nursing was predominantly a male domain as women were considered too delicate to care for severely injured men.

During the Crimean War, the War Office did permit a party of nurses, led by Florence Nightingale, to care for troops in Scutari. This move was viewed as an experiment by the War Office, and despite the myths that have surrounded the Nightingale legend, it did not fully endorse a commitment to female nursing until after the Boer War. Nightingale had, however, provided the initial breakthrough necessary for the formation and expansion of a military nursing service. A grateful British public had also set up a charity, and this Nightingale Fund was used to establish a military nurse training school at Netley and a civilian nurse training school at St Thomas' Hospital, London. Neither training school, however, fully incorporated Nightingale's own ideas with regard to the art of nursing. Nightingale had founded skilled nursing on the ranks, customs and traditions of the British Army, but civilian nurse training schools only adopted the features inherent in the military system, which would result in the formation of a compliant workforce. The military values incorporated into what became known as the Nightingale system centred on a sense of duty, self-sacrifice, discipline and respect for authority. Nightingale also recognised the importance of an 'officer class' nurse who would provide nursing leadership, but this feature of the military framework was overlooked in the civilian nursing field.

Yet, although the paramilitary Nightingale structure had linked nursing to military authority, this structure did not challenge sexual divisions of labour. Nurses remained subordinate to male physicians, and the profession continued to include middle-class notions of femininity, religious philanthropy and elements of domestic service alongside its military value system. However, long hours, petty restrictions and compulsory living-in arrangements all conspired to depress recruitment figures. This situation was compounded by excessive discipline procedures. Within the hierarchy of nursing frameworks, the matron ruled supreme and some were apt to rule their nurses in the manner of malevolent despots. The potential for some women to oppress other women, particularly the young and impressionable probationer nurses, had not escaped the attention of the Lady with the Lamp. Writing in 1878, Nightingale noted:

My views are exceedingly altered as to the supremacy of the Matron. It did very well for me whose fault is subserviency and civility. It does ill for Matrons whose fault is the love of power and lawlessness towards medical and other authorities and for Matronships where there is not a strong intelligent administration with power and duties running parallel to the Matrons.

Broaching the subject again in 1878, Nightingale cast more doubts with regard to matriarchal authority:

> I am not so sure now that nursing should be so entirely in the Matron's hands, now we [The Nightingale Fund] have no dominance over her. We have recommended people lately who ought not to be within a mile of a hospital.*

Military and civilian nursing fields were by now inextricably linked, and an Army Council initiative that was put forward to the humanitarian organisations of the British Red Cross Society and the Order of St John Ambulance Brigade in 1909 strengthened these ties. The initiative effectively enabled these voluntary humanitarian bodies to train VADs in order to supplement both military and civilian nursing services during a time of war. This arrangement was welcomed by some medical professionals and denounced as an attempt to dilute nurse-training establishments by others. Certainly by 1914 the British nursing services were politically divided between those who believed that nurse status should rest on the prestige and elitism of some training hospitals and those who advocated the need for a common standard of training and state recognition by means of state registration. The latter view eventually gained the most support. It is also worth noting that the drive for nurse registration was closely associated with the suffrage movement; many women believed that if they were prepared to join the military and make a vital contribution to the war effort, then surely they should get state recognition in terms of the right to vote and the right to assume registered nurse status once their training was complete. Yet the government clearly demonstrated that, particularly in a time of war, barely trained VAD nurses could easily swamp both military and civilian hospitals and

---

* These quotes are taken from *Notes on Nursing* by Florence Nightingale quoted in Baly, M., *Florence Nightingale and the Nursing Legacy* (1986) p. 181.

undermine all arguments for lengthy standard professional training programmes.

In reality, the Nightingale system had ossified, and when the Nurse Registration Act finally came into being in 1919, it did not produce uniform standards of training or adequate professional leadership. Politically, civilian nurses remained fragmented, and failure to agree on policy formation resulted in government intervention and the creation of a General Nursing Council. Significantly, with their failure to reach a political consensus, British nurses had engineered their own downfall and handed over control of their profession to government departments, which merely wanted to staff the hospitals as economically as possible.

British military nurses fared better than their civilian counterparts. They were not disbanded in 1918 like other female military units, and the Queen Alexandra's Imperial Military Nursing Service (QAIMNS) gradually established their own training schemes. In 1941 registered military nurses were awarded commissioned officer status and in 1945 became the Queen Alexandra's Royal Army Nursing Corps (QARANC).

For the purposes of this book, however, it is pertinent to recall how nurses were viewed by the Order of St John Ambulance in the late nineteenth and early twentieth century, a time when, rather outrageously, nurses' uniforms were allowed to be 2in above the ground:

A nurse must always be modest, but never prudish. If she remembers how high and holy the vocation of a nurse is (and it is a vocation, whether adopted for a life-time or for a single illness) if she is absorbed in her work and really anxious for the welfare of those under her care, she will be able to do many things for them from which in other circumstances she might shrink; for many things which would otherwise be repugnant are in serious illness done as matters of routine. But all this can be done without the slightest loss of modesty.

Modesty of mind and modesty of speech should never be lost … Great self-control is necessary and a determination to accept all duties of her calling with patience and good temper. Intelligence and good temper are also requisite. To be a good nurse all domestic duties must be thoroughly understood not necessarily to do them, but to ensure they are properly done.*

Eager to play their part on the international stage, from 1914 onwards trained nursing sisters entered the ranks of the military in large numbers. In addition, young women from all sections of society flocked to be trained as VADs. Most of these were then deployed in casualty clearing stations and base hospitals, where they cared for sick and wounded Allied troops. Despite their training, however, none of these women were prepared for the overwhelming stench of gas gangrene and trench foot, or for the gasping lungs of the men who had succumbed to the effects of mustard gas. The nightly screaming terrors of severely shell-shocked soldiers also alarmed the new recruits. In many instances nurses could do little but comfort a soldier as he was dying; before the discovery of penicillin and the widespread use of antibiotics, soldiers frequently died of their wounds as sepsis set in and continued unabated. Indeed, with regard to sepsis and fevers in particular, good nursing techniques often dictated whether or not a patient lived or died. Undoubtedly in some instances, recovery depended on the immune systems of the individuals concerned, but infection control, the use of various inhalations, poultices and sterile dressing techniques all combined to aid healing.

Undoubtedly, nursing at base hospitals during the First World War was not for the faint-hearted, and some nurses, faced with the appalling carnage and shocking wounds, simply gave up

---

* Quote from 'Volunteering for Service – Caroline Mulryne', St John Historical Society Proceedings, VOL.X., 1998, p. 9.

during the first six months of their deployment. Those who remained, however, fought their own quiet war against suffering and sickness with dignified compassion. Many of these nurses were from the higher echelons of society. They were brought up in a world of gentility, more accustomed to deportment lessons and taking afternoon tea than dealing with the mutilated and shattered bodies of injured soldiers. Yet they rapidly became resilient, determined and resourceful women who forged deeply moving and poignant relationships with their patients and other members of staff, establishing a camaraderie which was to last the war and beyond.

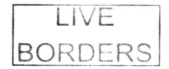

LIVE
BORDERS

I

Work began on the St John Ambulance Brigade Hospital in April 1915, the same month that Germany launched the first large-scale gas attack during an offensive near Ypres. It was the ninth month of the war, and so far events had not gone according to plan. The British had already suffered a humiliating defeat at Mons, and one in six of the 90,000 troops of the British Expeditionary Force in France were severely injured. Tented field hospitals, hastily erected in preparation for the wounded, were inundated with thousands of casualties before they were ready to receive them. Temporary dressing stations took the strain in most cases, with medical staff patching up the wounded as best they could. Amid the chaos and confusion, stretcher-bearers worked flat out, tirelessly moving soldiers away from the bloody carnage of battlefields, towards safety and some semblance of civilisation. Despite concerted efforts, however, some of the severely wounded were left to die where they had fallen. There were numerous failings in terms of transport, supplies and communication links, but more importantly the retreat at Mons had revealed glaring inadequacies in Allied medical care.

By supplementing British military medical services, the humanitarian efforts of the British Red Cross and Order of St John of Jerusalem attempted to improve this situation by supplying field ambulance units, trained medical staff and wound dressings. The greatest contribution made by the Order, however, was undoubtedly the establishment of St John's. It was designed and constructed by Messrs Humphreys of Knightsbridge London and, for its time, was a state-of-the-art institution. The

War Office had chosen the site well, near main railway sidings and north of a cluster of Allied base hospitals. Not far from the Somme, it lay eastwards of the main road between Étaples and Bolougne on the River Canche estuary. Less than a mile from the coast, the hospital was surrounded by undulating sand dunes, towering poplar trees and patches of swampy marshland. Beyond this area, the French landscape was dominated by beautiful rolling countryside. Miles of peaceful-looking meadows were as far as the eye could see, separated by neatly trimmed hedgerows adorned with colourful profusions of wild flowers: scenery that gave no hint of the further bloody battles to come.

When completed, St John's was the best-equipped medical establishment within the British Expeditionary Force. An American medical officer who toured the hospital declared, 'It is the best institution of its kind,' prophetically announcing that, 'this will become known as the Somme hospital'. The cost of maintaining each hospital bed was estimated to be about £100 a year. The twelve districts of the Order had raised in excess of £40,000 by the spring of 1915 and continued their successful fund-raising efforts throughout the war. Fund-raising and other public relations events were initiated and supervised by senior members of the Order. These included the grand prior, HRH the Duke of Connaught; the director of the ambulance department, Earl of Ranfurly; secretary general, Colonel Sir Herbert Perrot; lady superintendent in chief, Lady Ethel Perrot (Sir Herbert's wife); surgeon in chief, Mr Edmond Owen*; and chief commissioner of the brigade, Colonel Sir James Clark. The latter became the first commanding officer (CO) of St John's.

Colonel Clark had previously served in the Boer War, with Edinburgh and East Scotland Hospital at Norval's Point,

---

*   Mr Edmond Owen was appointed surgeon in chief in 1905 but died unexpectedly in 1915. His daughter, Cynthia Owen, served at the hospital as a VAD from 24 October 1915. Mr Owen was replaced as surgeon in chief by Sir William Bennett.

and was appointed chief commissioner of the brigade in 1911. An upright, thoughtful, intelligent medical man, with an unswerving attention to detail and devotion to duty, Clark embraced his new position as CO with considerable enthusiasm. According to his diary, he left England for Étaples on 22 July 1915, catching the 2 p.m. train from London's Victoria station and arriving in Boulogne at 6.35 p.m. He took control of St John's the following day and, under his expert guidance, buildings were cleaned, equipped and prepared to receive the sick and wounded. This process was not all plain sailing, however. Clark recorded in his diary:

> During the setting up of the hospital, the engine and dynamo for the x-ray machine and the operating theatres could not be traced. It had not, apparently, been landed at Boulogne. Stewart Gordon was sent to England to trace its movements and speed up its arrival.

Clark was also unhappy about the mortuary buildings. For ease of patient transfer the mortuary block was originally located very near to the wards. Concerned about the impact this positioning may have on the morale of his patients, Clark announced that it was quite unseemly to house the dead so close to the living. Therefore, on his instructions the mortuary was moved as far away from the wards as possible and a small cubicle nearby was turned into a makeshift chapel.

In the coming days, hospital departments, treatment rooms and wards began to take shape; as Clark noted with some satisfaction, the latter were particularly airy and attractive: 'The wards present a pleasing picture with their beds each covered with a grey quilt decorated in the centre with the badge of the Order in black and white.'

During August 1915 Clark spent much of his time giving various dignitaries guided tours of the hospital and assigning duties to his newly appointed medical and nursing staff. He had a clear vision of how his hospital would be run, reminding staff on a daily basis that Almighty God and sound Christian principles needed to be placed at the centre of their humanitarian service. The first church parade was held on 1 August, and services of thanksgiving were held every Sunday. Everyone was given ample access to Christian worship. Motivated by his religious fervour and humanitarian convictions, Clark was determined that his hospital would be the best in the region. Staff of the highest calibre had been recruited on six-month contracts; these could only be renewed if work was of a suitably high standard. Clark knew for certain that in the coming months his staff would be tested to their limits. Long hours, overwhelming workloads and numerous frustrations would take their toll. Keyed-up emotions and frayed tempers would undoubtedly surface from time to time. Thus, in an effort to pre-empt these problems and maintain staff morale, he established football and cricket teams, gymnastics and chess clubs, debating societies, a choir and a drama club.

Once content with the buildings, grounds and staff, Clark turned his attention to the more specific medical challenges posed by modern warfare. From the late nineteenth century onwards, the most prominent feature of warfare had been its ability to destroy the barriers between civilian and military life. Improvements in weapons technology, the building of railways and other communication systems, and the rise of industrial complexes all combined to restructure methods of warfare and medical practice. Furthermore, civilian welfare reforms were often initiated with military goals in mind. For example, the Liberal welfare reforms of 1906–14 were enacted because many men who had volunteered for service in the Boer War were medically unfit.

Nevertheless, in addition to highlighting the dubious fitness levels of recruits, the Boer War had provided military medical officers with valuable battlefield experience. Wounds that were inflicted on the sandy veldt of South Africa, however, were a far cry from the suppurating wounds of the Western Front. Almost all of the latter were infected with an *anaerobic bacillus*, which caused gas gangrene, a product of trenches swamped with manure. The foul stench of this condition permeated nearly every ward, and doctors were helpless to prevent its spread. They would cut away diseased tissue, but this failed to have any impact. In cases where limbs were affected amputations sometimes saved lives, but more often than not injured soldiers still succumbed to the toxic effects of the *bacillus*. Not surprisingly, a steep rise in the number of fatalities amongst previously fit and healthy young men prompted a certain amount of disquiet within medical circles. As one young surgeon confided to his journal, 'the men are dying at an alarming rate and there is nothing we can do'.

Fully aware of this appalling situation, Clark was astute enough to realise that newly emerging medical problems could only be overcome by research and experimentation. He formed a medical society on 18 August, and all medical officers in the Étaples region were eligible to join. On 1 September he reported that 'a very full meeting of the Étaples Medical Society has taken place'. Henceforth, he argued, members would need to initiate medical innovation and experimentation. They would have a God-given opportunity to not only be of service to their patients but also to make a phenomenal contribution to physiology, surgery and neurology. The Director of Gas Services, C.H. Foulkes, also shared Clark's view, pointing out that 'We have in the theatre of war itself a vast experimental ground ... Human beings provide the material for these experiments on both sides of no man's land.'

As scientists began to view the laboratory as a battlefield, military officials began to view the battlefield as a laboratory. In the meantime, physiologists back in Britain were busy carving out a niche for themselves as expert advisors to the government and the military, alongside industrial and business experts. These medical–industrial relationships intensified as new methods of warfare both prompted and accelerated research programmes. Dissemination of research findings through medical societies ensured that Colonel Clark, along with his contemporaries working on the Western Front, quickly became pioneers of surgical and medical practice. But theirs was a quiet war, fought in difficult circumstances with tenacity and perseverance. Significantly, it was also a war that could only be won with the help of skilled nurses.

Sitting at her large wooden desk in a rather chaotic-looking office, the newly appointed matron of the Brigade Hospital, Constance Elizabeth Todd, was under no illusion as to who would be at the forefront of this medical war. Nurses of all kinds, from all backgrounds, would be needed to provide excellent bedside care. Their practical skills, keen observations and tender ministrations would be needed in abundance. Almost buried under an assortment of paperwork, matron had been busy writing ward routines, rules, regulations and protocols for wound treatments since her arrival on the 11 August. Assistant matron Mabel Adeline Chittock had travelled with her to Étaples and was subsequently occupied with ward and treatment room inspections. Both women had trained at Guy's Hospital, London, and were renowned as indomitable, determined characters. Matron, originally from Yorkshire, had trained between 1904 and 1907, whilst her Norwich-born assistant trained between 1900 and 1903. Tall and stick thin, with delicate facial features, pale blue eyes and light brown hair, matron possessed a wiry energy. Mabel Chittock had a handsome, rather than pretty, face and was a large, well-built lady, with broad shoulders and a gentle smile. These women were very close friends and worked extremely well together. They even had nicknames for each other. In private, matron referred to Mabel Chittock simply as Chitty, and the latter referred to matron as Toddy. Three trained nursing sisters, Willis, MacMalon and Smith, had also arrived by this point. Further batches of nurses arrived in six drafts between 1 September and 22 October.

Matron welcomed each batch of nurses with a brisk tour of the hospital buildings and an induction speech, which she could recite from memory. Laying down firm ground rules, she would look fiercely at new recruits with her steely pale blue eyes, stating in a suitably sombre tone:

Nurses are not allowed to wear make-up or jewellery. You are to look smart and presentable at all times. You are to polish your shoes, buckles and badges to the Glory of God. You are expected to say Grace before every meal, prayers will be said on the wards at the start and the end of the day. Remember that as a representative of this hospital, you are expected to behave in a dignified, ladylike appropriate manner both on and off duty. You are not to wear civilian clothes under any circumstances, nor must you make any alterations to your uniform unless permission is given by myself or by my assistant matron. Be aware in the coming weeks that every patient thinks that he falls a little bit in love with his nurse. This is transitory however, you will discover that most men have womenfolk of their own back home. Similarly, nurses often mistake emotions of pity and sympathy for their patients with that of being in love. This is particularly true of young nurses who have had little or no experience of life before coming here. Make no mistake! I will not tolerate any romantic or clandestine associations between my nurses and their patients. It is of the utmost importance that you work to the very best of your ability. Any problems should be reported to me at once. The wellbeing of our patients is our overriding priority. Nevertheless I am also here to ensure the wellbeing of my nurses.

Matron's fierceness had totally subsided by the end of her speech, and she smiled kindly towards her nurses, with a twinkle in her eyes. After all, she wanted to earn their trust as well as their respect. This smile did not always have the desired effect. Most trained nursing sisters had heard similar speeches before and simply nodded their approval when appropriate to do so; whereas barely trained Voluntary Aid Detachment (VAD) nurses were terrified of Matron and quaking in their boots on their first day of service. With an average age of 23, these nervous new recruits to the nursing profession spent most of their time coming to terms with homesickness and the inadequacies of their training. Their VAD manual outlined basic training as follows:

> First Aid (annual requalification); map reading; hospital work; reception; diets; sanitation and improvisation of materials. Nurse training can progress from basic requirements to more advanced nursing on military surgical wards where volunteers may have to deal with more serious wounds.

Certainly the majority of VADs had worked for three months in a British military hospital before embarking for France. Not all, however, had advanced to dealing with more serious wounds. Lily Fielding, with untamed, wavy auburn hair and dark green eyes, was one such VAD, now trying to make herself at home in a purpose-built nurses' block full of other volunteers. Amidst the neatly made beds, white enamel jugs and small round basins, she foraged in her suitcase for toiletries and pulled out small framed photographs of her family. Tearful goodbyes to her stoical parents were already a fading memory, and she was consoled by the thought that her elder siblings were already serving on the Western Front. Her tall, strappingly built brother, William, worked as a stretcher-bearer in the Royal Army Medical Corps (RAMC), while her sister, Agnes, a trained nurse, worked in a military base hospital a few miles away. Their presence seemed almost tangible. As strange as it may seem, her homesickness was rapidly squashed by an extraordinary buzz of collective excitement. Young vibrant women surrounded her chattering together, exchanging personal stories, discussing their expectations and laughing at each other's jokes. With an abundance of energy and enthusiasm they were in the process of turning the unfamiliar into the familiar. They tried on their uniforms, giggling at the frumpiness of long black wash dresses, unbecoming white caps and aprons and clumpy black shoes. Along with their uniforms, they had all received hard oblong bars of brown Windsor soap, which smelt of a combination of spices and citrus fruit. It was a smell that would dominate dormitory life for the next few years. There was also a mountain of carbolic soap stacked forlornly in the corner of each nurses' block. This was to be used against infestations of head and body lice. Lights out at 9.35 p.m. brought an abrupt end to the chatter and clatter, though some girls were too excited to sleep. They simply tossed and turned until the trumpet sound of reveille heralded the morning scramble for washes and breakfast.

The nurses had reasonably expected their first patients to be injured or sick soldiers. This was not the case. About a third of the 141 RAMC orderlies had reacted very badly to their typhoid inoculations. Wracked with griping abdominal pains, vomiting yellow bile at frequent intervals and suffering from high fevers, they became the first occupants of the pristine hospital beds. Matron did her best to comfort these unexpected patients by informing them that their immunity against typhoid would be wonderfully high and long lasting. Green at the gills, the men were unconvinced.

The first few days of September signalled a period of intense preparation. Finishing touches were made to wards and large supplies of food were delivered. Final coats of paint were applied to window ledges and door frames, and outdoor sheds were stocked to the brim with general stores. Operating theatres and laboratories were functional, and cleaning-up parties were assigned to each block. Colonel Clark pounded the hospital corridors casting a critical eye over completed buildings. He then congratulated his staff on their hard work.

Yet a few problems persisted, and on 3 September Clark confided in his logbook, 'Torrential rain during the night.

Some leaks – chiefly where the electrician has used nails. Heavy rain all day.'

These minor glitches, however, did not delay the opening of the hospital. The following evening, the commanding officer wrote in his logbook in bold ink, 'Notified the authorities that the hospital is now ready to receive patients.'

Back in the nurses' block, Lily Fielding lay on her bed, nervous and full of self-doubt. Reaching into her bedside locker, she pulled out a letter from her sister, Agnes, and began reading:

> Your average British Tommy is a cheerful stoical sort of chap, who tries to make jokes even in the most appalling of circumstances. He is truly the most wonderful person to nurse, appreciative of everything you do for him and often more concerned for the welfare of others than for his own wellbeing.

Folding the letter carefully, Lily placed it under her pillow, closing her eyes as she did so. Soon she would learn the truth of her sister's words.

2

At 11.30 p.m. on 7 September, the first convoy of battle-weary patients arrived at the Brigade Hospital. First came the walking wounded, with heads, legs and arms covered with soiled bandages, splints and slings, bedraggled and grimy, and carrying small parcels of meagre belongings. With deep fatigue lines etched into their muddy weather-beaten faces and eyes dulled by pain, they shuffled and stumbled, many limping, into the hospital triage area. Those with severe injuries were carefully carried in by stretcher-bearers. In total, this convoy consisted of fifty-seven soldiers, all of whom had been involved in skirmishes near Loos. The commanding officer recorded in his logbook that thirty of these men were sick and twenty-seven were wounded. It was important to make this distinction on admission, primarily to ascertain which soldiers needed to be barrier nursed to prevent the spread of infection but also to record which, if any, would be entitled to a disability pension after the war. Those who were injured by friendly fire or by accident, for instance, could not subsequently claim any disability pension, regardless of the severity of their injuries. Soldiers rendered disabled by illness were also prevented from making any claim for compensation.

Severely wounded men were usually carried off the battlefields by RAMC stretcher-bearers, often as the battle was still raging. If there was a temporary lull in firing and conditions permitted, first aid could be administered on the battlefield and in the trenches; but the main aim of stretcher-bearers was to transport the wounded rapidly to a place of relative safety and the nearest first-aid post. However, some of the injured were forced by circumstance to make their own way to first-aid posts. Often this involved a journey of several miles on foot, under the cover of night. First-aid posts were discreetly hidden in the undergrowth, small copses, ruined houses or hastily made dugouts, yet it was here, in rudimentary makeshift huts, that the sick and injured received initial treatment. Subsequently, these patients were transported by horse or handcarts to dressing stations or field ambulance units. Further treatment was administered at this stage if necessary, and medical particulars were written down and attached to each patient's uniform. They were then taken by motor ambulances to a clearing hospital, where the injuries were assessed by medical officers in greater detail. Those patients deemed fit to travel were sent back to Britain by hospital ship, whilst those who required urgent attention and further monitoring were sent by hospital train to a base hospital near Boulogne. This whole process of medical treatment and assessment could take hours, days or weeks. Thus by the time muddied and bloodied soldiers reached the pristine white sheets, fluffy pillows and proper mattresses of their hospital beds, they had all but abandoned hope of ever experiencing such heavenly comforts.

According to the commanding officer's logbook, the first patients at the Brigade Hospital were all efficiently assessed, washed and bedded down by 1.30 a.m. Later that same day, he performed two serious operations: one an amputation of the thigh, another for a perforating wound of the knee. As the nurses gathered for their first proper shift, they said prayers before listening to the sister's report. For young VADs, hospital language was mystifying. According to Sister Margaret Ballance, who was in charge of O ward, there were a number of patients who were suffering from DAH, which stood for disordered action of the heart. Then there were NYDs, or not yet diagnosed patients; patients with GSWs had gunshot wounds; PUOs had pyrexias (high temperatures) of unknown origin; and DILs were patients on the dangerously ill list.

Sister Ballance also stated that a group of three soldiers at the far end of the ward were 'completely batty!'

Lily felt sure that she would never remember all these abbreviations, but a young, slightly plump, cheerful Irish nurse named Bessie Trimble assured her that such things would become second nature to her eventually. For Bessie, nursing at the Brigade Hospital was very much a family affair, since her cheerful, stoical father, Major Charles Trimble (later Colonel), was deputy commanding officer. Fortunately for Lily, Bessie appointed herself as her guide, friend and confidante. As they cleaned and tidied lockers, gave out food trays, rolled bandages, took temperatures and assisted with dressings and medications, they swapped personal stories and joked about the quirky natures of some orderlies.

The patients were amiable, and it was hard to judge how much pain they were in. When asked how they were feeling they would invariably reply, 'nothing much wrong with me, Sister' or 'mustn't grumble, miss' or 'I'm feeling chipper today and make no mistake about it'. The amputee patient, however, was very anxious, and he beckoned Bessie over to his bed. He was convinced that he could still feel his left ankle and calf, even though he had been told that his leg had been amputated. Bessie was a marvel: she pulled up a chair and took hold of his hand, stroking it gently as she spoke in soothing tones. Carefully and slowly, she explained a condition known as 'phantom limb syndrome' whereby the nerves in the leg continued to transmit false impulses to the brain. 'You will experience it for a few days at least,' she assured him. 'Sometimes, it continues for weeks, but it will pass eventually and your brain will adjust to the amputation.' The patient, a sturdy young man with tousled brown hair, a well-groomed moustache and deep brown eyes, looked unconvinced but was somewhat mollified by Bessie's gentle approach and obvious concern. 'My name is Raymond,' he said quietly. Bessie smiled and withdrew slowly from his bed. 'Well Raymond, we will do our best to take care of you while you are with us. Soon we will bring round some beef tea. I am sure that will build your strength up.'

The CO had ordered that all men should have 1 pint of beef tea and ¼lb of bread on their first day following admission. Working on the premise that many of the men had not received a good meal or adequate nourishment for some days or weeks before coming into hospital, he believed that strong beef tea was essential for building up the constitution of his patients. In the cookhouse the overpowering aroma of beef tea was a constant reminder of the ebb and flow of hospital admissions. Fresh, nutritious food was produced daily and made a welcome change to the soldiers' usual meal of 'bully beef', which consisted mainly of fat and gristle. Any leftovers were distributed to the poor of Étaples.

On 15 September a flag of the Order of St John of Jerusalem was raised above the hospital in honour of a visit from the chairman of the Joint War Committee and members of the Red Cross Commission from Boulogne. This visit from what the orderlies called 'Top Brass' sent all staff into a frenzy of cleaning, polishing and tidying. Matron inspected all wards, dressing rooms, nurses' quarters, the cookhouse, laundry rooms and departments. Thankfully the visit went ahead without any hitches, except for a strange smell that emanated from one of the drains. A middle-aged orderly named Bert, who had a strong Cockney accent, had taken to pouring large batches of tea leaves down the same drain several times a day. A combination of tea leaves and heavy rains had created a blockage. Bert was duly reprimanded and given the task of unblocking the offending drain.

By the end of September, sisters, nurses, doctors and orderlies had adjusted to the rhythm of ward routines and leisure periods. Patients were nursed cheerfully and with a greater degree of confidence than had been apparent earlier in the month. Unable, or unwilling, to make certain distinctions between qualified nurses and VADs, patients tended to call all nurses 'Sister'.

Those with sensitive egos took time to describe the various nurse trainings to patients, who usually smiled amiably and reverted to calling every female 'Sister' again. It was, as Sister Margaret Ballance said, 'a bit of a lost cause'.

Some of the patients were now improving in leaps and bounds, and there had only been one death that first month: a gunner named Stuart, who had been riddled with gas gangrene. A few injured soldiers had been able to return to their duties, and the commanding officer established a recreational committee for those who were convalescing. A small library was constructed near the cloakrooms, and officers in particular were encouraged to read, paint, sketch and play cards. All wards were now full, and the list of advice, official notices and instructions for both staff and patients seemed to grow with each passing day. The War Office was particularly concerned with the fact that male staff and recovering patients might fraternise with dubious women who were intent on assisting the enemy. Commanding Officer James Clark took these concerns very seriously, to the extent that he insisted on reading out loud a War Office memo on the subject to all patients in every ward, and to all male staff members. The memo read as follows:

Soldiers are warned that the enemy is very crafty and energetic in obtaining information of numbers, formation and movements of the British Army. Such is their redoubtable system of espionage that nobody can detect for certain who is in their employ. It is therefore of the utmost importance to refrain from giving any sort of information by writing or in conversation. It may always be passed on or repeated in the hearing of a spy.

A favourite dodge of the Germans is to employ women of easy virtue to wheedle out of us bits of information. Intercourse with unknown women should be rigorously avoided. These women will probably endeavour to make you without your meaning to do so, give them information.

Remember that the smallest bit of information – the name
of a regiment, the brigade or division it forms part of, the
names of places where the regiment has been, or is stationed
on the front, the time of arrival of a unit or a reinforcement
– carefully pieced together will afford valuable information
to your enemy. Keep all mention of such things out of your
letters and conversation and help beat the enemy.

This speech prompted a few mutterings under ward blankets,
mostly along the lines of 'chance would be a fine thing' and
'where on earth would we find a woman of easy virtue'. But
the commanding officer remained solemn and poker-faced.
Nursing staff stood to attention around piping hot ward stoves,
expressionless for a few minutes and springing into action
only when Colonel Clark had disappeared from their sight.
Clattering cutlery on supper trays, the squeaky wheels of
medicine trolleys and bustling VADs bent on tidying patients'
bedside lockers for the umpteenth time, soon usurped grim
warnings about espionage. Moreover, it is not clear how big a
threat such potential liaisons between military men and local
prostitutes posed to British Army security. From a military
medical standpoint, these relationships were already dangerous
because they encouraged the spread of venereal disease; for this
reason alone, some French cafés were designated as being 'out
of bounds' for British soldiers, including officers.

For most of the nursing staff, whose virtue was beyond
reproach, the idea that prostitutes might be lying in wait to lure
their patients or fellow staff members into dens of iniquity was
nothing short of a moral outrage. Such women were considered
to be teetering on the brink of hell fire and brimstone at the
very least. Military nurses, trained or otherwise, were never
allowed out with a man without a chaperone, even for the
briefest of walks. The tippets that were worn by members of
the Queen Alexandra's Imperial Military Nursing Service were
designed to hide a nurse's sexuality, as were the frumpy dresses

and pinafores of VADs, and the blanket coverings provided by floor-length capes. In their off-duty periods, St John's nurses were encouraged to walk on nearby St Cecile Plage beach, where the air was bracing and invigorating. There was also an infrequent bus service into Étaples village, but in an effort to protect them from raucous, drunken soldiers on leave, nurses were discouraged from venturing out in this direction. On rare occasions, such as someone's birthday, a group of six or more nurses would walk into the village and take tea in one of the quaint cafés. They were provided with a list of respectable establishments. There were also guidelines about how a nurse should take care of herself, which were pinned on the entrance doors to the nurses' quarters.

A Nurses' duty to herself.
A skilful nurse is careful of her health.

Cleanliness:
The necessity for personal cleanliness as to body, hair, teeth etc., – is too apparent to require discussion. The need for professional cleanliness is equally important because in infectious diseases the chief danger is the taking of food with infected hands.

Appetite:
Health depends on a good digestion and the latter is controlled by appetite. An inviting tray of food in pleasant surroundings is as necessary for the nurse as for the patient.

Rest:
Sleep and rest are essential to health. The nurse must therefore, have a separate bedroom – well aired and well ventilated. Further, dressing gown and slippers must be available for emergency night work.

Exercise:
Regular exercise is conducive to health. The minimum
period off-duty per day should be spent in the open air.

Food:
The nurse must never go on duty tired and hungry. If she
does, and if she is attending to an infectious disease, then she
will incur unfair and increased dangers of infection. No food
should be taken in the sick room.

Uniform:
The apron should be clean and ample in size. The boots
or shoes must be polished every day. The dress needs to be
no higher than an inch off the ground, this regulation is to
ensure modesty and to avoid the mud that may be present
on duck boards and pathways.

Guidelines were often flouted of course, and many a nurse
skipped breakfast in preference for an extra twenty minutes
in bed, whilst some spent more time preening in front of the
mirrors than others. Then there were those who, by their very
nature, routinely left everything to the last minute, hurriedly
pinning hair up under starched caps as they scooted down
corridors en route to their wards.

Every morning Matron inspected both wards and nursing
staff. Nothing escaped her eagle eyes. A counterpane crease
slightly off centre, a jug placed too near the edge of a locker, a
flower vase with stale water, a misspelt name card, a stove that
needed stoking, a nurse with unpolished shoes: all would be
noted by Matron with an air of delicate distaste. Once inspection
was over, the relief was palpable and routine work resumed. Lily
dutifully followed Sister Margaret Ballance during her first few
days, like a puppy dog glued to its owner's feet. Slim, fair-haired
Sister Ballance was in charge of one of the busy medical wards.
As far as Lily could ascertain, trained nurses seemed as though

they were always doing something important with glass dressing trolleys and lengths of rubber hose, whilst VADs were occupied with more mundane tasks such as giving out hot drinks and endlessly cleaning lockers. On her first day Lily had broken two thermometers, one medicine glass and lost a patient's false teeth. The latter had fallen down the sluice and took some considerable effort to retrieve. Now, however, she was feeling less like a fish out of water. Bessie had helped her, both on and off duty, to understand the mysteries of hospital life, and she was beginning to feel more confident. On 24 October another VAD, named Cynthia Owen, arrived; her father, Edmund Owen, had been surgeon in chief of the Brigade. He had died suddenly, and Cynthia was still in a state of bereavement. Encouraged by her mother to become a VAD, she fervently believed that by coming to nurse in Étaples she was, in some way, continuing her father's work. Cynthia was a shy, awkward young woman with large, deep-set blue eyes, high cheekbones and porcelain skin. Bessie naturally extended her nurturing once again to the new recruit, whilst Lily realised, with some anxiety, that she was now considered to be experienced.

Bessie, Lily and Cynthia were later joined on O ward by a Canadian VAD nurse named Emma Mieville who was reserved and artistic by nature. Sister Ballance and her junior sisters, Bertha Smith and Annie Bain, coaxed and chivvied their trained and untrained nurses until O ward ran with ease, like clockwork. Orderlies scurried around underpinning routines when necessary and dealing with most of the more unpleasant jobs such as the laying out of dead bodies. Nurses were only expected to lay out the dead if the patient died during the night. More intimate tasks such as shaving 'men's privates' in preparation for theatre were also undertaken by orderlies.

Significantly for medical and nursing staff, the character of injuries continually changed, posing new challenges and accelerating experimental treatments. In 1914 when trenches were shallow, soldiers were more likely to suffer from leg and foot injuries. By October 1915 deeper, sunken square trenches protected feet and legs from gunshot wounds, and head wounds became more prevalent. This shift in changing wound sites and characteristics prompted new approaches to medical care. Of particular concern was the growing presence of gunshot wounds consisting of multiple shrapnel shards that became embedded in the brain. Numerous neurosurgical operations resulted in failure because it was, for some time, impossible to retrieve small pieces of shrapnel. A lunchtime conversation between medical men, however, revolutionised cranial surgery. This group of medical men, which included American neurologist Dr Harvey Cushing, theorised that by using a nail as a probe into the brain and then attaching a magnet, shrapnel slithers and balls would be drawn out by attraction to the magnet. Dr Cushing, who possessed specialist expertise, worked at several hospitals in France, including the Brigade Hospital. He described the first successful operation conducted with a nail and a magnet in his detailed journal:

> Several unsuccessful trials this morning to extract shell fragment by aid of magnet from the brain of poor Lafourcode. We had tried every possible thing in our own cabinet and in those of lower floors without success. Finally, while I was at lunch, Boothby hit upon precisely what was needed in the shape of a large wire nail about 6 inches long, the point of which he had carefully rounded off.
>
> Well there was the usual crowd in the X-ray room and approaching corridor, and much excitement when we let the nail slide by gravity into the central mechanism of smiling Lafourcode; for at no time did he have any pressure symptoms, and all of these procedures were of course without an anaesthetic.
>
> While the X-ray plate was being developed to see whether the nail and missile were in contact, who should drop in but Albert Kocher with a friend from Berne; and then shortly

a card was sent in by Tom Perry's friend Salomon Reinach, *Membre de l'Institut*, author of the *History of Religions* and much else.

So altogether we traipsed into the first-floor operation room, where Cutler mightily brings up the magnet and slowly we extract the nail – and then – there was nothing on it! Suppressed sighs and groans. I tried again very carefully – with same result. More sighs and people began to go out. A third time – nothing. By this time I began to grumble: 'Never saw anything of this kind pulled off with such a crowd. Hoodooed ourselves from the start. Should have had an X-ray made when the man first entered the hospital.' The usual thing, as when one begins to scold his golf ball.

I had just taken off my gloves and put the nail down; but then – let's try just once more! I slipped the brutal thing again down the track, 3 and ½ inches to the base of his brain, and again Cutler gingerly swung the big magnet down and made contact. The current was switched on and as before we slowly drew out the nail – and there it was, the little fragment of rough steel hanging on to its tip! Much emotion on all sides – especially on the part of A. Kocher and Salomon, Reinach both of whom could hardly bear it.

Experimental surgery became the norm as new weapons technology inflicted increasingly fearsome injuries. Wound therapies became more complex and treatments more invasive. Yet amongst these changing medical scenarios there was considerable respect for the somewhat reserved British approach to medical administration. Dr Cushing noted in his journal:

This is truly a man sized job, in the midst of which the Britisher stops for tea, and everyone, down to the Tommy – has time to shave; and it's this taking–it–quietly, that possibly enables them to see things through with some measure of composure.

There was also a robust camaraderie that permeated hospital life, particularly amongst nursing staff. By mid-November Bessie, Lily, Emma and Cynthia had cemented their own intimate friendship circle. They shared their daily ups and downs, confided secrets in each other and talked of their future aspirations. Bessie was already feeling a romantic attachment towards a certain Captain Alan Brunwin, who worked in the cardiology department. Brunwin was a handsome, clean-shaven young man, with straight brown hair and hazel eyes. Bessie was teased mercilessly and blushed whenever his name was mentioned. She insisted that her attraction to Brunwin was merely an idle flirtation, but her friends knew better. Lily was yet to feel any attachment for anyone or anything other than her work, though she enjoyed reading romantic novels in her off-duty periods. Emma spent her off duty doing the most remarkable sketches of landscapes and the hospital. While Cynthia was gradually emerging from her grief and fancied herself as an amateur botanist, picking up leaves and obscure plants, referencing and pressing them. Sister Ballance, meanwhile, seemed to spend her off-duty hours writing lengthy letters home; she sometimes shared this time with sisters from other wards. She had a good relationship with her junior sister Bertha Smith, but they worked opposite shifts. Night sisters also formed their own friendship networks. Moreover, friendships once made were rarely disturbed or broken.

Off-duty conversations varied. In the doctors' mess for instance, new operation techniques, medical discoveries and ongoing research programmes usually dominated discourse. In this sense they were never really off duty. At least twice a week, however, they ventured further afield either in the commanding officer's car to fetch supplies or in a motor ambulance. During these times they recorded the changing seasons and beautiful landscapes, dotted by craters, trenches and barbed wire. Nurses usually discussed more personal subjects, such as family, friends and spiritual beliefs. Indeed, in the autumn of 1915, the latter subject dominated thinking and debate in nurses' quarters. Many of their patients were adamant they had seen spiritual beings on the battlefields. Some claimed to have seen the Angel of Mons. Others had seen visions of Agincourt Bowmen. According to patients, these apparitions usually occurred immediately before a battle. Not surprisingly, nurses were quite perplexed as sensible, logical-thinking men recounted such seemingly far-fetched stories. Descriptions and timings of ghostly beings were compared at length in dormitories as nurses drank their evening cocoa, with some giving credence to these visions and others dismissing them as total nonsense. One thing was certain, however: descriptions of apparitions were remarkably similar in all cases and seen by men who were not prone to hysteria. Opinion on this subject remained divided throughout the war, but to severely injured men, many of whom had lost close friends in battle, spiritual apparitions provided some small semblance of comfort.

3

By the end of October 1915 it became apparent that an increasing number of soldiers were being admitted to hospital suffering from disordered action of the heart (DAH). Complaints of chest pain, dizziness, palpitations, tiredness and breathlessness were more commonplace, and DAH eventually became the third most common cause of medical discharge. Some of these unfortunate soldiers had suffered from rheumatic fever in their childhood, which had left them with weak heart valves. Others had heart problems because of bacterial infections or as a result of advanced venereal disease. Within the British Expeditionary Force, thanks to an Irish physician named Dr John Elder Macllwaine, the Brigade Hospital was the only medical establishment with a cardiograph machine. Dr Macllwaine, a scholarly looking man with steel-rimmed glasses, had bought his own cardiograph machine whilst working in Belfast at the Royal Victoria hospital. In 1915 he then transported it to the Brigade Hospital, where it was installed next to the X-ray department. Electro-cardiograms (ECGs) quickly became an important diagnostic tool, and as the workload increased, Captain Alan Brunwin was employed as Macllwaine's assistant.

Within medical circles generally, the value of ECGs was heavily disputed, with some doctors claiming that they were of little or no use. The cardiograph at this stage was rudimentary. Electrodes were attached to the patient and tracing leads were taken for each photographic plate. The galvanometer used an exceptionally fine fibre to register every heartbeat. All soldiers suspected of having heart problems were subjected to cardiograms along with those over the age of 40. Dr Macllwaine was responsible for the supervision of three medical wards in addition to his role within the cardiograph department.*

Medical assessment of heart disorders, however, was also influenced by central government research programmes. These in turn were motivated by economic considerations. A soldier classified as suffering from DAH, for instance, could expect to spend nearly six months in hospital, whereas if his symptoms could be described as 'effort syndrome' then the time spent in hospital could be reduced to six weeks. This reduction in hospitalisation saved the government about £50,000 a year. Consequently, tremendous pressure was exerted on medical staff to re-evaluate symptoms and downplay their significance. The concept of 'effort syndrome' was introduced in an attempt to divert attention away from anatomical heart defects and disease, towards a condition that could be deemed far less sinister in nature. According to government advice, a soldier's complaints of pain, giddiness and fatigue needed to be reclassified as being relatively normal manifestations of effort, rather than being symptomatic of a more serious underlying heart condition. Furthermore, this advice suggested emphasis needed to focus on overall heart function rather than pre-existing heart defects. The government-backed Medical Research Council also argued that ECGs were of limited value in determining levels of heart abnormality. Henceforth, both civilian and military doctors were encouraged to ignore heart abnormalities in favour of measuring overall performance. Yet despite this economically driven reclassification of heart symptoms, statistics recorded in the Brigade Hospital logbooks clearly indicate that Dr Macllwaine did not comply with this new trend. There was no mention of effort syndrome in any of his notes. Inpatients with heart

---

* Dr Macllwaine returned to civilian medical practice in July 1917 but died in tragic circumstances. After the war his eyesight began to fail, and he was convinced that he had a malignant tumour. Fearing a slow and painful decline, on 6 August 1930, at the age of 56, Dr Macllwaine took his own life.

abnormalities numbered 1,045, of which 1,031 were diagnosed with DAH. The majority of these patients had diseased heart valves. MacIlwaine proposed a regime of graduated exercise to improve heart function, which was implemented in convalescent wings. Soldiers who responded well to exercise eventually returned to the front line, those who did not were medically discharged and sent back to England.

MacIlwaine also conducted his own research, making detailed case notes of all his patients, comparing their diagnoses and ECG results. He and his assistant, Alan Brunwin, meticulously documented patients' presenting symptoms along with their clinical appearances and medical examinations. Together they produced several medical papers on the subject of ECGs, which confirmed both diagnostic and monitoring benefits of cardiograms.

By November 1915, however, Captain Alan Brunwin had other matters of the heart on his mind. He had fallen for the charm and beauty of Bessie Trimble. Eager to court her in the proper fashion, he had asked his colleagues in the officers' mess for advice. Head surgeon Major Maynard Smith, renowned for his booming voice, had none to offer, claiming that women remained one of life's most peculiar mysteries. Luckily Major Thomas Houston from the pathology lab had more to say on the subject, stating with some confidence that most women liked to be listened to and they all seemed to like flowers. This was not much to go on, but Alan was determined to make an effort. He very deliberately bumped into Bessie in the corridor one morning and asked her if she would accompany him into Étaples to take tea. Bessie had smiled encouragingly and said that she would be delighted to take tea with him, but it would have to be the following day, since this was her only off-duty period for the week. Arranging to meet her at 2.45 p.m., Alan congratulated himself for getting over the first hurdle. He set out that evening to find some wild flowers, only to discover that these were distinctly lacking in November.

On the day of their assignation, Bessie awoke at 5.30 a.m. with the trumpet sounding reveille in the nearby parade ground. Gathering her washbag, she walked briskly to the washrooms and filled a white enamel basin with cool water. She was looking forward to spending time with her captain. Until recently they had only exchanged shy glances and the odd greeting as they passed each other in the corridor. This afternoon they would hopefully discover a bit more about each other. It had taken her some considerable time to persuade Lily to act as chaperone, for she was engrossed in a Jane Austen novel that her sister had sent earlier in the week. Bessie told Lily that watching a romance blossoming at first hand must surely be preferable to simply reading about it. Lily was not sure. Acting as a gooseberry was never an attractive proposition. Bessie promised her some cake and a pot of proper tea, but this had little impact. Finally Bessie appealed to Lily by stating that a time might come when their roles would be reversed; then Lily would need a chaperone. Lily did not think this situation would happen any time soon, but if romance should happen to come her way then it would be nice to be able to call in a favour.

Everything was arranged for the afternoon of 16 November; when Bessie pulled back her curtains after her wash, however, she was alarmed to discover that the hospital and grounds were covered by a thick blanket of snow. Thrown temporarily into a panic, she woke Lily and quickly blurted out how everything would probably be cancelled and she would not be able to meet Alan again for at least ten days. Was this a sign that their relationship was doomed? Lily rubbed her eyes and peeped out of the window. It was not like her friend to be so dramatic. She pressed her face against the glass, momentarily transfixed by the beauty of distant stark trees covered in white. Ignoring the practical considerations that such a dramatic turn in the weather presented – such as how to get back and forth to Étaples, whether or not any tea shops would be open or whether further snow falls would arrive and leave them completely stranded – Lily clasped her hands in glee. Infused with optimism underpinned by a firm conviction that snow added a delightful sense of romance to the whole day, she chivvied her despondent friend along the corridor for breakfast. Bessie had lost her appetite, but Lily remained positive and ate like a horse. They were both required to work that morning before enjoying their off-duty. While Bessie fretted Lily teased, laughingly informing her friend that coping with inclement weather would be the first test of her captain's ardour.

In the administration block, Colonel Clark sat writing in his logbook: 'Snow – very heavy during the night.' He was concerned about how such a turn in the weather would affect heating bills. Costs were rising steadily as a result of wartime inflation. Coke already cost 23s a ton and coal 31s 6d a ton. Furthermore, bad weather conditions could prevent deliveries, not only of fuel but also of vital medical supplies such as medicines, dressings and lotions. These worries weighed heavily on his mind.

Captain Brunwin was also preoccupied with the weather. Determined to meet up with his sweetheart, he made concerted efforts to secure transport to and from Étaples. After much persuasion he managed to bribe an RAMC orderly, who was driving a motor ambulance to Étaples after lunch to collect food supplies. This was not ideal, because the driver was expected to return by a certain time to unload his goods. But it was better than nothing. Besides which, the orderly had stated with a wink, with further bribing he could be persuaded to 'have a puncture on the way back, if you see what I mean Sir'. Bribes needed to be in the form of alcohol, cigarettes, biscuits, jam or other foodstuffs, since these substances were difficult to obtain.

At the appointed time Brunwin picked up Bessie and Lily in the motor ambulance. He had kindly brought along a copy of *The Times* for Lily to alleviate her boredom whilst he and Bessie chatted. Conversation was quite stilted en route, however, partly because the ambulance driver kept interrupting their discussions. Teashops in Étaples were impromptu establishments known as *estaminets*. They were often located in the front living rooms of private houses, but they did have cakes and authentic tea and coffee. If an officer had access to reliable transport he could travel further afield, where it was possible to find high-quality restaurants. Bus routes were mainly used for transporting staff and luggage, and certain cafés were out of bounds as Colonel Clark's logbook reveals:

> Memo DAQMG
>
> The motor bus service between Etaples and Camiers is primarily for the use of Nursing Sisters returning to their hospitals.
>
> Café L'Usine between Camiers and Dannes, and Café Lekey at Camiers is out of bounds.
>
> Café De L'Union Rue de Rosomel is now in bounds.

Cafés could be designated out of bounds for a variety of reasons: the possibility of spies lurking in their midst, the existence of some infectious disease in the area or a lack of food quality. As Alan, Bessie and Lily arrived in Étaples, there were two cafés open, both with very few customers. They chose the more secluded of the two and hurriedly entered through a large oak door, keen to get out of the cold. Lily sat at a corner table, hiding behind the newspaper to afford her friend some privacy. Bessie and Alan were escorted by a plump waitress to a window table and gradually began to relax. Alan talked about his ambitions and prospects at work. As one would expect, he was extremely knowledgeable about medicine and war. He told her that recent battles at Loos had been very disappointing. British casualties numbered 48,367 during the primary thrust, with 10,880 further casualties sustained in follow-up attacks. He then proceeded to outline the problems of treating Indian casualties, particularly those from Gurka regiments, since apparently they point-blank refused to have amputations even if desperately needed.

Their religious convictions dictated that they should be whole in body in order to be transfigured properly after death. Alan was also concerned that infectious diseases were weakening military personnel. Currently there were at least 9,000 victims of typhoid, and in the first two weeks of November alone there had been at least 300 cases recorded each day. Fortunately most British troops had been vaccinated so there were only a handful of typhoid cases amongst some of the unvaccinated soldiers. Bessie, who was used to discussing such things with her father, knew some of this information already, but she hung on to his every word regardless. He encouraged her to talk about her work, but she was reluctant to do so. She had spent the entire morning establishing the number of constipated patients and considered this to be a highly unladylike topic for conversation. Instead, she diverted him on to the weather … a safe subject if ever there was one. Time flew by rapidly. An hour and a half seemed to have gone in the blink of an eye. Trudging out, trying to make fresh footprints in the snow, they laughed and threw snowballs at each other. A perfect gentleman, Alan kissed Bessie's hand as he helped her into the ambulance once more. Lily insisted on making her own way into the ambulance, handing back the newspaper as she did so. The return journey was bumpy and quite treacherous. Further snow had fallen, drifting in some areas and making driving difficult. The sun had gone down in the grey overcast sky and the temperature was plummeting. Wrapped in long woollen overcoats, faces flushed from throwing snow, Alan and Bessie resembled excited children. The date had gone well. Lily, despite her reservations, had also enjoyed the outing.

Snow lay thick on the ground for a few days and seemed to bring out the child in everyone. A scattering of snowmen dotted the hospital grounds and some orderlies had instigated an igloo competition with a packet of biscuits for the winner. Amidst all this frivolity, on 26 November Colonel Clark made another of his grim announcements:

Attention is drawn to the fact that measles is prevalent at present in the neighbourhood of Etaples. Every precaution should be taken to prevent, as far as possible, intercourse between the British inhabitants of this Base, and the French population. Attention is particularly drawn to the risk of infection being conveyed by clothes sent to local laundresses for washing.

Later that day Lily confided in Cynthia that she thought Colonel Clark was obsessed with preventing intercourse at all costs. All his warnings seemed to mention the subject, as though people were 'at it' all the time. Nevertheless, dire warnings about measles were well founded. This was a life-threatening disease, which in severe cases resulted in blindness, deafness, seizures and encephalopathy. Furthermore, by 2 December Lily, Cynthia and Bessie were covered in a measles rash. Along with sister Ryecroft and nurse Dillion from D ward, they were sent to No. 24 general hospital to be barrier nursed in darkened rooms. Nurses from all base hospitals succumbed to measles at an alarming rate, but most of them survived unscathed. Cynthia was left with a slight deafness in her right ear, whereas pasty-faced sister Ryecroft had experienced burst ear drums in both ears; fortunately this had not affected her hearing. Lily had initially seen the illness as an opportunity to read more romance stories, and she was most put out when a sister told her that because measles potentially affected the eyesight, she should not read for at least three weeks. Bessie, upset that she was not allowed to see Alan, consoled herself with the thought that both she and her friends should at least be well by Christmas.

To some extent, hospital routine had been undermined by the measles epidemic. Nursing sisters who remained in good health were required to work far longer hours, with some having no off-duty hours for over a month. Company orders also recorded a few changes in personnel in the run up to Christmas festivities. Matron Todd had been given leave to visit

England because her father was very sick. Major Trimble took over Colonel Clark's position while he was on leave; Captain Hope took charge of the surgical division of the hospital during Major Maynard Smith's absence on leave, and Sister Gould relieved Sister MacMahon as night superintendent.

Major Charles Trimble, as acting commanding officer, began to organise carol concerts and musical plays, which he hoped would entertain both staff and patients. All staff and patients were also given Christmas postcards to send home to relatives. Writing company orders, Trimble observed strict censorship rules, stating, 'There is no objection to the following being written on Field Service post cards: *A Merry Christmas and a Happy New Year.*' He added, despondently, 'I don't think that many of the men will know or care what day it is.'

Amongst the overall administration duties, Trimble was expected to deal with a number of petty incidents as they arose. For instance, on 15 December he recorded:

> A charge of riding a bicycle without a light has been made by one of the military police against Pt Johnson number 61292. Pt Johnson of St John Company – ran into the policeman who was also riding a bicycle. Damage was done to the policeman's bicycle. I dealt with the charge and admonished Johnson. I advised him to pay the cost of the damage when known.

Trimble was also expected to run the hospital efficiently regardless of staffing levels. This efficiency was often put to the test, such as on 17 December when medical authorities decided to issue evacuation notices to certain hospital commanding officers to check the speed of their evacuation procedures. Trimble recorded:

> An evacuation notice was received at 8.55 to evacuate at 9.45 at siding – wholly impossible to meet demand. However,

patients were coming into the receiving block at 9.30 and whole move was completed in 55 minutes. I consider this to be quite smart work, but nothing of importance happened.

Evacuation times, which were influenced by efficiency levels generally, staff turnover rates, numbers and types of patients, placement of tents or huts, availability of ward orderlies and their respective strength and build, knowledge of instruction manuals and frequency of practice drills, varied between hospitals. Company orders at the Brigade Hospital were as follows:

Evacuation Arrangements
Select Non Commissioned Officers and men from A or B party – but not from the party doing convoy duty on previous night.

Cooks and sanitary squad not to be used for evacuation duty in early morning.

If ward orderlies are needed use smallest number possible. The Non Commissioned Officer in charge must dismiss them to the wards at the earliest moment.

One sergeant required to take charge of stretcher cases. One Non Commissioned Officer (night N.C.O. if available) for walking cases. One Corporal for trollies and ten orderlies for every twelve to twenty stretchers, including two tall, strong, orderlies for loading wagons.

These evacuation procedures were crystal clear and worked well in the absence of any further problems. If evacuation orders were received at the same time as incoming wounded, however, procedures were not so straightforward. Logbooks record that a steady flow of patients were evacuated on a regular basis in order to make room for more seriously wounded men. These evacuations often took place at night and were recorded alongside other noteworthy news. For example, the logbook entry for 20 December 1915 reveals that:

At 5.30am 16 stretcher cases and five sitting cases were evacuated. Sergeant Carr and Private Beaumont of R.A.M.C. were admitted to hospital. Quartermaster off duty with a boil on his leg.

21st December as follows:

Convoy of wounded men arrived at 12.10 – 89 stretcher cases. One officer evacuated to Boulogne – special authority from A.D.M.S. (Captain Mason A.S.C.)

These almost daily evacuations were implemented at the discretion of medical officers; they were not the result of orders from above. Higher medical authorities would only issue full-scale evacuation orders either to test efficiency levels in this respect, or because they had received intelligence reports indicating that certain hospitals were at risk from enemy attacks. In many instances, however, hospitals were attacked without warning.

4

A few days before Christmas, Lily managed to visit her sister, Agnes, in Boulogne. They shared tea, sandwiches and cake in a nurses' club, which had been formed and funded by a Mrs Robertson Eustace. The establishment was essentially a rest home for military nurses; with a welcoming bathroom, comfortable beds, elegant tea rooms and a library, it provided much needed respite from the rigours of nursing duties. Lily was full of admiration for her sister's temporary luxurious surroundings. These included sumptuous gold-coloured window drapes, plump embroidered cushions, gilt-edged landscape paintings and ostentatious chandeliers. Round mahogany tables were covered with exquisite white lace tablecloths, and tea was served in dainty little china cups. As Lily continued to survey the scene, Agnes, who looked like an older version of her sister, cheerfully informed her of all the other luxuries the club had to offer: a hot bath whenever you felt like one, appetising meals and beds with soft feather pillows. Books could be taken out of the library at any time during the day, as long as they were returned a week later. Lily felt as though she had momentarily stepped into one of Jane Austen's novels, instead of the nurses' club at 4 Rue Cozin Boulogne. Agnes, laughing at her sister's wonderment, reminded her that she had to be back at work by Christmas Eve.

Nurses were allocated respite periods if they had worked excessive hours or if they were recovering from illness. Agnes had worked for nearly three months without any off-duty time. Furthermore, in addition to working her day shifts she had often been required to work during the night. By the time she entered the nurses' club she had not had a proper night's sleep in over sixteen weeks. There were nights when, with swollen aching feet and her head pounding with exhaustion, she had almost cried with tiredness. Her hands, red raw, were chapped from a combination of bitterly cold weather and a shortage of gloves with which to do saltwater wound irrigations. Unlike Lily, who worked and slept in purpose-built wooden-hutted quarters, Agnes had only tented accommodation, which by comparison offered little shelter from biting winds and severe frosts. Her time at the club, however, had given her a new lease of life, and being able to meet with her sister had further lifted her spirits. Following their delightful tea, they exchanged Christmas gifts, each giving a sincere promise to keep them wrapped until Christmas Day. Then affectionate hugs, smiles and kisses were suddenly replaced by tinges of sadness and loss, as Lily boarded an overcrowded bus bound for Étaples.

On the wards, Christmas 1915 was a subdued affair. Orderlies had done their best to ensure that every ward had a small fir tree decorated with cones and sweets. In the cookhouse turkeys of various sizes adorned the racks and smells of plum pudding filled the air. A stream of brown paper packages arrived daily from Britain, containing all sorts of gifts: knitted balaclavas, socks, scarves, gloves, Christmas cakes, biscuits, pots of jam, sweets, condensed milk and cigarettes, usually Woodbines, Navy Cut or Gold Flakes. According to the post office, over 250,000 parcels were sent to the Western Front in the months leading up to Christmas. In addition, bales of tobacco, cigarettes and matches were sent to the hospital from various charitable organisations. Black Cat cigarettes were also very popular, since packets of these cigarettes usually contained a free English-to-French phrase book.

On Christmas Eve, small parties of doctors, nurses and orderlies toured the wards, singing Christmas carols. They asked if anyone had a request for a special song, but few of the men responded. Most were detached, listless, homesick and in pain.

When the time came to eat Christmas dinner many of them could not even eat properly. Amongst the ranks neglect of oral hygiene was rife. Although a set of reasonable teeth were a prerequisite for enlistment, a combination of poor diet and chain smoking had rotted their teeth and gums. Over a third of inpatients required some form of dental treatment, their mouths a disgusting mix of nicotine-stained teeth, ulcerating flesh and inflamed gums. Trimble inspected these mouths personally and claimed that they were in an appalling state. Captain Coe, the fastidious dental officer for base units, concluded:

> The general condition of the teeth of patients is deplorably bad. With the exception of men recruited from the upper, and to a lesser extent the middle classes, and members of the Colonial forces there is almost an entire absence of appreciation of clean mouths and care of teeth – numbers of men frankly stating that they had never used a tooth brush in their lives.

Given this lack of oral hygiene, it was not surprising that the majority of men ended up having some or all of their teeth extracted.

Elsewhere in France, new dental treatments were being pioneered by the likes of Dr Hayes, who introduced new and amazing methods of jaw realignment along with thorough dental hygiene programmes. He worked primarily with soldiers who had lost half of their faces in battle, carefully reconstructing and remoulding their jaws and mouths into recognisable facial features. At the Brigade Hospital, however, dental treatment was limited. As the acting commanding officer acknowledged:

> Colonel Carr Adams called to see what assistance our dentist could gain for general work to be sent from the convalescent camp. He pointed out that he was only required to do such work as would fit a man for the fighting line as soon as

was possible. He said that dentists should communicate with
the Officer Commanding at the convalescent camp – and
tell him how many he could attend to each day, and settle
him an allowance.

Basic dental care was given to all inpatients who required it,
but for those who had several rotting teeth, extractions were
the only option. Gargling with saltwater was encouraged, but
a lack of teeth severely limited types of food intake. There was
no question at this stage of a patient being fitted with false
teeth, since moulding, constructing and fitting new teeth was
considered to be too expensive and time consuming.

In addition to oral hygiene problems, skin conditions were
also prevalent, the majority of men being riddled with lice,
fleas and scabies. Most had rubbed whale oil into their feet to
prevent trench foot, but this was not always effective. Ill-fitting
boots caused swollen ankles, deformed toes and painful blisters.
Other men had suffered severe frost bite and lost toes as a result.
Soldiers were required on occasions to stand for weeks at a time,
knee deep in mud and freezing cold water; these circumstances
resulted in poor circulation to the feet, leaving them blue and
numb. The stench of taking a soldier's boots off on admission
to hospital could be overpowering. It was also difficult to strip
them of their uniforms on arrival. Caked with blood, mud,
horse manure and rats' urine, uniforms were usually cut off with
scissors and scalpels.

Fragments of material had often been burnt into wound
sites and had to be carefully removed with tweezers. Men faced
with this prospect would bite into their pillows, knuckles white
from gripping on to bed frames, rather than utter a scream
of pain. It was commonplace for a soldier to be admitted to
hospital with multiple wounds, and the excruciating agonies
associated with wound debridement and irrigations were a daily
occurrence. In stoical silence these soldiers suffered, not only
from the searing physical pain of their wounds but also from

the vivid, traumatic memories of battle. Most had witnessed shocking scenes of barbarity and destruction. Tales abounded of horses being blown clean up into trees, their innards draping across withered winter branches. Patients described men for whom there had been no hope, those with completely exposed abdomens and severe head wounds, limbs blown feet away by the impact of shell explosions and those so peppered with shrapnel they could no longer draw breath.

Then there were those who had been present during gas attacks. Dr Harvey Cushing recorded their experiences in his journal:

> When we got back to the ambulances, the air was full of tales of asphyxiating gas which the Germans had turned loose – but it is difficult to get a straight story. A huge, low lying greenish cloud of smoke with a yellowish top began to roll down from the German trenches, fanned by a steady easterly wind. At the same time there was a terrifically heavy bombardment. The smoke was suffocating and smelled to some like ether and sulphur, to another like a thousand sulphur matches, to still another like burning rosin. Only sixty men out of a thousand survived the attack.
>
> Later I saw a number of recently 'gassed' cases – two of them still conscious, but gasping, livid and about to die, and I hope they didn't have long to wait poor chaps.
>
> Then we saw many of the severely gassed men who had come in this morning – a terrible business – one man as blue as a sailor's serge, simply pouring out with every cough a thick albuminous secretion, and too busy fighting for air to bother much about anything else – a most horrible form of death for a strong man.

Images such as these were impossible to erase from the minds of those who had witnessed them. Some lay catatonic between starched white bed sheets, unaware of their surroundings, too dazed from battle fatigue to care whether they lived or died. Others, more alert, surveyed each other with empathy, registering the suffering of their brothers in arms. One who was blind had formed a friendship with another who was deaf; each dependent on the other's senses, they insisted they were placed in neighbouring beds. A few, though maimed and mutilated, were on the point of recovering.

Yet despite the horrendous array of wounds, manifestations of shell shock, lingering effects of gas attacks, fevers and disease, Major Trimble attempted to generate some semblance of Christmas spirit. This was a monumental task and a report compiled by the hospital secretary stated emphatically:

> We had about three hundred and seventy patients in hospital and I think those who were able to, enjoyed themselves; although there were many, unfortunately, to whom it was anything but a day of pleasure.

In addition to the gifts that were received from relatives, the Order of St John supplied patients with a pipe or cigarettes. Patients also received extra food rations, a small tot of brandy, a bottle of beer or stout, or a soft drink. Gifts for the medical and nursing staff were provided by The Ladies Committee of the Order. Medical Officers were given engraved match boxes and nursing sisters received a silver buckle for their belts. Nurses were also given an 'Arms of the Order' brooch by Major Trimble. Christmas Day began with prayers, and Holy Communion was celebrated on every ward. Local almoners visited each patient, discussing their needs and offering help where they were able. Christmas dinner was served at midday followed by more prayers. A 'lucky dip' tub full of gifts was a feature on all wards, and staff gave a musical concert designed to improve morale.

All medical staff, nurses and orderlies not absent on leave took part in Christmas festivities. They sat by patients' bedsides encouraging them to sing along with Christmas carols and other songs. They held their patients' hands when homesickness threatened to overwhelm them, read out their letters and cards from home, and helped to feed those with facial injuries. At times such as these the British 'Tommy' would often reveal a rather dark humour. For example, when Lily gave a bottle of beer to a double amputee named Harry Hall, known as 'H' to his friends, he had smiled at her, saying, 'No more for me, Nurse, or I'll be legless.' Lily had returned his smile, but as she'd walked towards the kitchen to get him some barley water, tears had filled her eyes. Another young man, named Reginald, who had been operated on for severe abdominal injuries, winked as he told her that he couldn't have brandy, 'I haven't the stomach for it you see, Sister.'

When they were not making fun of their own wounds and circumstances, soldiers would spend a considerable amount of time inventing nicknames for individual staff members or groups. Surgeons and physicians with memorable mannerisms would be ridiculed relentlessly. For instance, there was a moustache twister, a nose wiper and a lopsided eyebrow raiser amongst the medical staff; VADs were called anything from 'Very Adorable Darlings' to 'Very Angry Despots'. Humour helped to lift morale and acted as an antidote to self-pity.

Major Trimble, acutely aware of morale levels, possessed an abundance of quick Irish wit. With jovial flare and relish he would spontaneously invent comical stories and jokes to entertain his men. His ability to conjure up humour at will, however, frequently masked his deeply reflective and spiritual nature. Indeed, there were times when responsibilities weighed heavily on his mind. Recently a bright, handsome young man from the Rifle Brigade had died from post-operative complications, and that very Christmas morning an officer who was convalescing had died unexpectedly in the officers' mess. For Trimble and others, these deaths cast a long shadow over Christmas festivities. Staff had said prayers for these men in a makeshift chapel, but there was no permanent chaplain to give comfort and spiritual guidance. A Reverend T.A. Lee had been temporarily appointed on 9 October, but his quarters were based in the Allied Forces hospital.* Furthermore, he was required to spend most of his time conducting funerals. By this stage, like a sinister, silent, slow-moving tidal wave, graves of the fallen were beginning to dominate the landscape.

As Christmas Day drew to a close, the day shift nursing staff retreated to their quarters. Lily had given her sister a small, wooden trinket box carved with delicate flower shapes for Christmas. One of the hospital orderlies had been a carpenter in civilian life and had made several decorative boxes to order. He made them in his off-duty time, using small tools such as a scalpel, and charged only a few francs. Each box was unique in design and big enough to store small items of jewellery or a nurse's hospital training badge. Agnes had given Lily a new novel entitled *The Wooing of Rosamund Fayre*. Written by Amy Roberta Ruck, who had shortened her name for publishing purposes to Berta Ruck, the romantic text appealed greatly to Lily. However, although eager to get started on her book, the atmosphere was not conducive to reading. Three new sisters had arrived on 22 December and they had brought with them lots of homemade Christmas treats. Sisters Margaret Freeman Rutherford, Victoria Hartwell and Ella Gordon Grant were fresh-faced, enthusiastic young women, all determined to share their special treats with fellow nurses. These included tiny plum puddings, star-shaped biscuits, little blocks of fudge, sugared almonds, butterscotch, almond toffee, peppermint creams in small boxes tied with red ribbon and an abundance of fruit-flavoured sugar drops. Exchanging gifts whilst enjoying these sugary delights, the sisters' mess and nurses' quarters were

---

* Eventually Reverend F.E. Gower was appointed as full-time chaplain, but Colonel Clark objected to his appointment on the grounds that he did not hold an army commission. Therefore, Reverend Gower was later replaced by Reverend C.H. Mylne, who remained as hospital chaplain for the duration.

buzzing with excitement for over an hour. Then, as tiredness set in, they prepared their beds for sleep. Before lights out, however, they all solemnly agreed that there was one important act they needed to perform: one of sincere remembrance. A few sisters had managed to secure small quantities of brandy from the dispensary, which they put into mugs of cocoa for everyone. With a small hand gesture from Margaret Ballance, the room fell eerily silent. Raising their mugs slowly in an act of sombre solidarity they proposed a Christmas toast to one of their own – a courageous nurse who had stated that she was happy to die for her country – Edith Louisa Cavell, an English nurse and heroine, who was executed by a German firing squad on 12 October 1915 for helping over 200 Allied soldiers to escape from German-occupied Belgium. As nurses sipped their brandy-laced cocoa, reflecting on Cavell's supreme sacrifice, the melancholy sound of the last post echoed through the cold night air.

5

Matron Todd, recently returned from compassionate leave, sat at her desk catching up with paperwork whilst listening to echoes of 'Auld Lang Syne'. A small party of nurses, orderlies and officers had gathered in a recreation tent to dance, drink punch and welcome in the New Year, but Matron was in no mood to celebrate. Huddled in her heavy woollen overcoat, grieving the loss of her father, she had decided to bury herself in work. Besides, the year 1916 was heralded not by a joyful peal of bells but by a sinister rumbling of exploding shells. Then, suddenly, the hospital was plunged into total darkness as Zeppelins droned loudly overhead. Matron abandoned her work and retreated to the sisters' mess, fumbling her way awkwardly through pitch-black rooms as she did so. Unable to sleep, fearing that patients might need to be evacuated at any moment, she thought about how she could improve the skills of her nursing sisters. As things stood, sisters were placed on a ward when they arrived, be it surgical, medical, urology or neurology etc., and there they remained for the duration of their contracts. Matron was convinced that this policy led to stagnation in terms of nursing care – a belief that things should be done as they had always been done. It fostered expertise in one field of nursing and virtual ignorance of another specialism. A preoccupation with this problem kept her awake for much of the night. Nevertheless, by morning Matron had reached a decision. The only way to improve matters was to introduce a rotation system, whereby sisters changed wards every three months. This way sisters would have experience on all wards and become more versatile as a result. The rationale behind

Matron's decision was quite simple – in case of injury or disease, a ward sister might need to be replaced at a moment's notice; if those replacements did not have the necessary experience, chaos could ensue and patients would suffer.

Matron announced her new policy in the sisters' mess at lunchtime on New Year's Day. It was greeted with enthusiasm by some and dismay by others. There were those who felt as though a rug was being pulled out from under their feet. Older sisters in particular did not relish change. They were comfortable in their existing roles and argued that their status would be threatened if they were placed in charge of unfamiliar wards. Furthermore, there was always a chance that an experienced VAD might have more knowledge of nursing practice on certain wards than those in charge – a situation that would surely undermine respect for nursing sisters. Matron acknowledged that there might be a few teething problems associated with her rotation scheme, but overall she was certain this policy would lead to improvements in patient care.

Working on the premise that soldiers' wounds and injuries were growing more frequent and complex by the day, Matron also ordered sisters to elevate the status of experienced VADs by instructing them in a variety of dressing techniques. Any VAD who had worked at the hospital since its opening in September 1915 was considered to be experienced. For Lily, this was something of a revelation: she was finally going to discover why bits of rubber tubing were so necessary for wound treatments.

Lily's curiosity was satisfied early one Monday morning, when a quiet pretty sister with soulful hazel eyes and dark hair, named Dora Little, asked for her help on the dressings round. Not knowing what to expect, Lily jumped at the opportunity. Once they arrived in the dressing station, Sister Little showed her how to make up a solution called Dakin's fluid. This solution needed to be made up as and when it was needed because it became unstable very quickly. Consisting of 0.4 per cent sodium hypochlorite and 4 per cent boric acid, Dakin's fluid

was simply a very weak bleach solution. Accompanying Sister
Little to the bedside, Lily was taught how to use the rubber
tube system to irrigate wounds, flooding them periodically
with Dakin's fluid, then using a stopcock system to drain them.
Lily quickly became adept at this technique, but she found
other aspects of dressing wounds to be extremely unpleasant.
It was a complete mystery to her how Sister Little remained so
cheerful when faced with such carnage on a daily basis. Trying
to mask her shock and pity, Lily first dressed the thigh wounds
of a young man named Percy Thomas. He was a chirpy sort of
fellow but watched Lily's face most intently as she worked. Like
many soldiers, he had sustained multiple injuries. The worst
of these was a very deep, wide thigh wound. Removing the
existing dressing delicately with sterile steel forceps made Lily
feel distinctly queasy. Percy's wound was badly infected. Gauze
and bandages were heavily stained with a mixture of coagulated
stale blood and suppurating green pus. When the old dressing
was eventually lifted out, much of his thigh bone and muscle
tissue was exposed. It was not a pleasant sight. Then, as she began
irrigating his wound, the stench of his rotting flesh combined
with bleach was almost overwhelming. Lily was determined not
to show her horror as the fluid ate away at the man's dead tissue,
exposing further glimpses of white thigh bone and lean muscle
tissue. When irrigation was complete his wound was once again
packed with gauze and bandaged securely. Sister Little assured
her that Percy's wound was improving by the day and looked far
better than it had the previous week. Lily found this statement
hard to believe, but she gave a reassuring smile to her patient.

Over the following days, Sister Dora Little, unassuming,
with a natural air of authority, imparted her knowledge and
wisdom to Lily in a gentle fashion. Whilst some sisters spoke
sharply or condescendingly to VADs, Dora adopted a soft tone
of voice. In her view, there were many intelligent VADs who
could be easily trained to do more complex tasks. To confine
these women to mundane work such as cleaning lockers and

dishing out cups of tea was quite simply a waste of resources. In one of their many discussions, Dora informed Lily about the raging medical debates that surrounded the treatment of wounds. A British bacteriologist named Sir Almroth Wright had conducted research in Boulogne, and by 1916 he began to attack the use of antiseptics in wound therapy. According to Wright, antiseptics destroyed not only bacteria but also phagocytes – white blood cells designed to eat away at bacteria. Wright advocated the use of hypertonic salt solution in wound irrigation since, according to his theory, this solution would stimulate the release of phagocytes, activating natural defence mechanisms. Wright's theory became known as a physiological approach to wound treatments and prompted considerable controversy. Research elsewhere, conducted by the French biologist and surgeon Alexis Carrel and an English chemist named Henry Drysdale Dakin, suggested that irrigation with a solution of buffered hypochlorite produced the best results.[*]

Lily was fascinated by Dora's knowledge and would often seek her out at meal times to hear her latest thoughts about nursing practice and medical debates. Not that Lily was allowed to eat at the same table as Dora or other nursing sisters. The nursing sisters had their own mess and dining quarters; VADs were confined to their own block. A strict hierarchy was maintained at all times. Lily had once made the mistake of walking up to a medical officer on a ward to tell him some information about one of his patients. Sister Annie Bain on

---

[*] Wound treatments were essentially 'a work in progress' throughout the war. Clinical trials initially endorsed the Carrel-Dakin treatment, and most hospitals adopted Dakin's fluid as the favoured method of wound irrigation. In later years, however, doubt was cast on the efficacy of Dakin's fluid as other more powerful treatments were introduced. Sir Almroth Wright was best known for his development of the anti-typhoid vaccine. He continued his work on immunology after the war, working alongside Professor Alexander Fleming, who discovered penicillin. In recent years Wright's work has been revisited by scientists eager to determine precisely how a person's natural defence mechanisms can be stimulated.

C ward had reacted as though the world was about to end: how could she even think that a mere VAD could approach a doctor in such a familiar way? All information about patients needed to be given to trained nursing staff, and then they would impart this information to medical staff if they thought it necessary. Lily thought this to be rather a long-winded process, but she did not make the same mistake again. However, she did want to learn as much as she could about nursing practice in order to help patients on her ward. Dora was in the habit of taking a brisk walk in the hospital grounds after mealtimes, and Lily would sometimes ask if she could join her. Impressed by her eagerness to learn, Dora would simply smile and nod her head. Sometimes they walked in silence, and other times they discussed the weather and the plants that were beginning to thrive in the hospital gardens. Birdsong often filled the air, and Dora was quite an expert at distinguishing different bird species. Most of the time, however, they talked about patients, not as individuals, since this would break strict confidentiality rules, but as groups of patients. Dora believed that the men needed to be out in the fresh air as much as possible; she was quite sure that being confined to a hospital ward for any length of time was detrimental to their health. Convalescent soldiers, particularly officers, were able to go out and about each day for a short while. Officers and other ranks even organised gymnastic displays and sports tournaments. Colonel Clark had resumed his position as commanding officer, and it was clear that he, like Dora, advocated fresh air as a boost to health. The latter, however, believed that doors and windows to wards needed to be flung open at every opportunity, if only to alleviate the smell of disinfectants.

Sometimes on ward rounds, other times as they walked in hospital grounds or as they took tea, Dora listened to medical officers discussing current issues in medical innovations. Occasionally she would hear them talking about lectures given at medical societies. Quiet and seemingly insignificant, Dora simply listened more than she spoke, acquiring snippets of information as and when she was able. Some of these snippets she would share with Lily or with her peer group in the sisters' mess. Occasionally doctors would discuss wider problems and issues, such as political changes on the home front and the state of war. There had been a heated debate quite recently between doctors who believed that Germans did not intentionally bomb hospitals and those who believed that Germans had no such reservations. As one doctor pointed out, Zeppelin raids on England had already damaged hospitals. He further argued that since, for ease of patient transfer, Allied base hospitals were usually located near railway lines, this geographical position made them easy targets for the enemy. After a few days of discourse on this matter, conversation drifted on to other subjects, and Dora was quite disappointed to learn that most doctors were against women's suffrage. Although not an outright feminist, Dora did think it was about time that women had more of a say in how things were run.

Lily had given women's suffrage very little thought until Dora questioned her about it during one of their walks. Cynthia and Emma had talked rather favourably about suffragettes, and her sister, Agnes, was sympathetic to their aims, but Lily was not enamoured. Involvement in women's protest movements and militant actions did not appeal to Lily one little bit. In fact, she had adopted Florence Nightingale's view on the subject. Before her death in 1910, Nightingale had acknowledged that society treated women unfairly, but she persuasively argued that women could never change things or improve their lot until they became economically independent. Nightingale was no supporter of women's suffrage and had openly declared that the vote was nowhere near as important for women as having access to their own money. However, by establishing nursing as a respectable profession in which women could move away from hearth and home, and earn their own money in the process, Nightingale arguably did more for women's liberation during her lifetime than the vote ever could. Both Agnes and Lily were ardent fans of this great lady and had read her book *Notes on Nursing* from cover to cover. Moreover, there was a courageous and idealistic element in all of Nightingale's endeavours that appealed to Lily's romantic nature. Agnes had sent her a copy of Nightingale's views about military nursing before she had volunteered as a VAD, and they had resonated in her mind. According to Nightingale, female military nursing could be likened to casting a stone on a pond, creating ripples of kindness which were far reaching and long lasting. These ripples reminded soldiers of their mothers, wives, daughters, sisters and sweethearts, of tender feminine comforts, of home and normality. When Lily felt tired, cold or homesick she remembered Nightingale's words and they strengthened her resolve.

Confessing these views and thoughts to her mentor as they walked by neatly trimmed lawns and budding shrubbery, Lily anxiously awaited her response. Dora agreed with Nightingale's assessment of women's needs and her view of military nursing but suggested that votes for women could well assume much greater importance in the future. Dora was an optimist and hopeful that women would gain the vote eventually because of their worth in society. The war offered women an opportunity to demonstrate their abilities, and this could be a turning point in women's history. Lily was not entirely convinced by Dora's optimism but nodded her head in agreement. Drizzly rain, rendered horizontal by a brisk wind, encouraged them both to curtail their walk at that point.

Back in the nurses' quarters there was much chattering about reported German atrocities. According to some of the orderlies, advancing German forces had used women and children as human shields. Stories abounded about shootings of hostages, raping of Belgian women, bombing of churches, gassing of whole villages, failure to respect white flags of surrender, the shooting of captured officers, and the poisoning of wells and other water supplies. How much of this talk was based on fact and how much on rumour, Lily could not tell. Bessie, who had heard them first hand from Alan, now her fiancé, gave credence to some of these reports. Alan believed that the story of poisoned water supplies, however, was probably a rumour, since contaminated water would affect German troops as well as Allied forces.

Alongside these dreadful accounts of atrocities were stories of narrow escapes and uplifting heroism. Men who had survived shelling because they had ducked their heads at appropriate moments or were carrying books in their breast pockets which had stopped a bullet in its tracks. Dr Harvey Cushing recorded some such cases in his journal:

> In our ward is a man who got off with a slight burn of the forearm when a German contact shell exploded near him, and yet many of his companions were killed. Another man had both bones of his forearm broken in a similar fashion without actually being hit, and yet his more distant companions suffered heavily from shrapnel. One man was blown into a tree and hung there for a long time by his trouser leg. Another was blown out of a trench and found the timing piece of a shell in the seat of his trousers. Many have barely escaped because they happened to be stooping when a shell exploded nearby. One artillery officer was knocked down three times in succession by shells landing only a metre or two away from him; he suffers from a severe nervous concussion – what the British call shell shock.
>
> A hammock stretcher has been devised which allows seriously wounded men to be promptly evacuated from the trenches without waiting till dark as has hitherto been necessary. They can be carried through the winding passages, only the hands of the bearers and poles of the stretchers being above the level of the trench when they come to make a turn.

Peculiar wounds seen:

An officer, hit in the trenches by an explosion of enemy hand grenade, had a small wound of entrance near the inner canthus of the right eye without special symptoms. An x-ray showed an un-deformed cartridge in the frontal lobe of the brain. This was extracted and it proved to be an intact French label cartridge! I give it up. He explains that the captured French ammunition, which of course does not fit the German Mauser rifles, is used with whatever else may be handy to fill hand grenades, now so murderously thrown about in trench fighting.

Lily listened intently to all rumours and stories but did not dwell on them. Friends often teased her about her reading material, but romance novels provided an essential form of escapism. Bessie had her captain, Emma had her drawing and Cynthia collected plants; Lily had her books. Nursing sisters also had their private passions, a few of them wrote poetry or belonged to a drama group, some listened to classical music or enjoyed singing in the hospital choir, while others had taken to bird watching or enjoyed long walks on St Plage beach. Everyone needed some kind of diversion, some semblance of life without war, a retreat into normality.

Spring was now in the air and the French countryside awash with a carpet of narcissus, wild violets, snowdrops and lilies of the valley. Sunshine interspersed with light showers of rain highlighted trees in bud and profusions of small anemones. Inviting woodlands, with their leafy walkways flanked by commanding beech trees, looked wonderfully peaceful and gave no hint of the blood-red landscape that was to come.

6

By March 1916 it was becoming more common for soldiers to be admitted with multiple wounds. There was also a dramatic increase in the number of soldiers admitted to the Brigade Hospital suffering from neurasthenia, otherwise known as shell shock. These soldiers frequently exhibited widespread body tremors with periodic muscle jerking. Usually their faces were transfixed with rigid expressions of terror and they lay unresponsive, virtually unconscious in their beds. With unblinking, glazed and protruding wide eyes, they seemed to be staring fixedly and uncomprehendingly into the distance at scenes that were so horrific they had rendered them senseless. Some uttered gibberish constantly, as though trying desperately to communicate some urgent thought or information. Any sudden loud noise – a dropped teacup for instance, or a loud voice – would prompt full-scale uncontrollable convulsions in these men. Then there were groups who were completely catatonic, unable to respond to any stimulus whatsoever. They were difficult to nurse, reluctant to eat or drink and incontinent. Moreover, since shell shock was a new phenomenon, it was difficult to diagnose and treat. Eventually labelled as NYDN (not yet diagnosed nervous), shell shock victims were initially placed in far corners of hospital wards in the hope that rest and gentle nursing would improve their condition.

Hitherto, small groups of men who were suffering in this way had been simply dismissed by sisters and medical staff as 'batty'. Growing numbers of such men, however, prompted a medical rethink about the causes and treatment of shell shock. To begin with doctors believed that shell shock had an organic cause. They surmised that men who were very close to loud exploding shells suffered from small haemorrhages in the brain, which rendered them semi-conscious and traumatised. Furthermore, post-mortem examinations of men who had died suffering from a combination of shell shock and gas attacks did indeed show small, multiple brain haemorrhages. However, the brains of shell-shocked men who had not been subjected to gas attacks did not show similar haemorrhages. When post-mortems failed to substantiate an organic theory of shell shock, doctors were at a loss as to how to treat the condition. Henceforth, patients suffering from shell shock were often accused of malingering.*

Medical staff at the Brigade Hospital treated shell shock patients in a non-judgemental way, with gentle compassion. This was not necessarily the case elsewhere. Suspected by many as feigning illness to avoid front-line duties, they were frequently ignored or left until last in terms of care. Moreover, military commanders in the field began to fear an epidemic of neurasthenia, believing that somehow men who displayed symptoms of a nervous disposition would pass on this condition to other troops. They further argued that men could easily mimic these symptoms in order to shirk their duties. Consequently, a variety of medical tests, which aimed to catch malingerers, were introduced.

Various assumptions were also made about the presence of shell shock in officers, compared to other ranks. The former, because of their elite upbringing and training, were above suspicion and therefore rarely accused of deliberate malingering. Yet shell shock in other ranks was considered to

---

*   Some wartime literature states that malingering and shell shock were one and the same thing. This was not the case. Nowadays shell shock is usually referred to as 'post-traumatic stress syndrome'. For further information on how shell shock was perceived between 1914 and 1918 please see 'Report of the Committee into "Shell-Shock"' (London, HMSO, 1922). See also Cooter, R. 'Malingering in Modernity: Psychological Scripts and Adversarial Encounters During the First World War' in *Medicine War and Modernity* (Sutton, 1998) pp.125–48.

be due to a lack of moral fibre. Thus the lower ranks were open to all types of accusations; supposedly their lack of breeding left them open to dire lapses in moral fortitude. These class distinctions affected the ways in which men were eventually treated for their neurasthenia. Officers were encouraged to rest, listen to music, paint landscapes, write poetry and read books. Relaxation and recuperation was the order of the day. Other ranks had no such tender treatment. Instead, they were subjected to extremely tortuous medical examinations, which were aimed at flushing out and exposing would be malingerers. Aversion therapies were used in an attempt to jolt men back to reality. Burning cigarettes were placed on their tongues and electric currents passed through their bodies. Both psychological and physiological examinations were devised to determine real from feigned illness. Medical officers were encouraged to become detectives in this respect, and those who were considered to be soft on malingerers were very quickly relieved of their positions. Yet the process of detecting malingerers posed considerable ethical problems for doctors, since it betrayed traditional, confidential doctor–patient relationships, viewed by many to be sacrosanct. Records of the Brigade Hospital, however, show that malingering was not necessarily synonymous with shell shock. According to the official book of company orders, the first case of malingering was detected on 9 December 1915: the commanding officer simply wrote, 'Prisoner sent to 24 General Hospital on suspicion of self-inflicting wounds.' Subsequent cases were few and far between, but malingering patients were primarily imprisoned for self-inflicted gunshot wounds rather than for displaying shell-shock symptoms.

Nevertheless, there was no doubt that malingering was on the increase, Dr Cushing noted:

Skulkers in ordinary wars simply lagged behind, whereas here the men must go into the trenches where a panic may seize them and where there is no officer's backs to keep your eye on and to follow where he may lead. These wounds appear to be particularly common among the Indians. In a recent convoy there were fifty wounds of the left hand, five of them among the whites and forty five among the Indian troops a disproportion too great to be a mere accident of figures.

The men, when questioned, explain that the top of the trench gets shot away by the enemy's fire and that they have to push the earth and sand bags back with their left hands. Powder stains, of course, would tell; but they have learned to interpose something – formerly a piece of wood, until splinters found in the palm were recognised as a tell-tale.

Cushing also recorded:

Three men who purposefully shot themselves through the hand were found out – not a difficult wound to recognise one would think. However, it is not always easy to spot a malingerer whether or not he bears a self-inflicted wound, and it is always possible that injustice may be done to one who gets sick or injured in some justifiable way.

Referred to by the men as 'swinging the lead', 'shamming' or 'skulking', malingering became almost an art form for men determined to escape the savagery of front-line service. Turpentine was used to create pus-like excretions, egg protein was added to urine to indicate kidney infections, and a wide variety of acidic solutions were ingested in the hope of causing jaundice. Some soldiers and sailors would inject their superficial wounds with pus from those suffering with venereal diseases or infected boils, and others would feign paralysis in legs or arms. They often shared or sold information (or 'tricks of the trade') and kept abreast of new medical technology. Indeed, the list of a malingerer's techniques was seemingly endless. Penalties for such behaviour, however, were severe, even fatal. Soldiers caught malingering would be court-martialled and sometimes executed.

The relatively low incidence of malingering at the Brigade Hospital was due largely to the fact that the hospital usually admitted the most serious cases. This practice resulted in a higher than average death rate but a much lower than average incidence of feigned injuries. A state-of-the-art pathology laboratory also played a part in this trend, since substance abuse and other attempts to mimic illness could be quickly exposed before admission. Major Thomas Houston and Captain John McLoy, who were both athletic men, were in charge of the pathology lab. Routine tasks included the analysis of blood samples and other bodily fluids, testing for gastrointestinal diseases, inoculations, blood transfusions, bacteriological tests, post-mortems and the distribution of antiseptic dressings. Houston and McLoy also provided adequate supplies of distilled water. Normal drinking water in this area was quite often cloudy because it was filtered through chalky ground.

Captain McLoy was also responsible for nearly all post-mortems, a task that became all too frequent as the war progressed. There were strict guidelines for the laying out of bodies after death. If a patient died in the day then orderlies would lay out the body; if a patient died in the night, however, a sister and VAD would undertake this work. According to nurses' handbooks, adherence to certain paperwork and protocols were extremely important:

Routine in ward in case of death of patient.

1   The sister informs medical officer in charge of ward, or in his absence the Orderly Officer.

2   The Medical Officer or Orderly Officer fills up the specially printed death labels. Particulars for these labels are to be taken from the diet sheet and not from any other forms on the head board.

NOTE – it is essential that the utmost care should be taken in filling up these labels.

3   One of the labels is tied firmly round the neck of the body.

4   The other label with all sheets from the head board and the brass tally are returned immediately to the Registrar's Office with a slip of paper giving the height and shoulder width of the body.

Important – remember to fill in a card of condolence for the deceased patient's relatives.

Cards of condolence contained words of sympathy and a photograph of the Brigade Hospital. Occasionally letters written by commanding officers would also be sent to relatives of the deceased.

Lily had only seen one dead body since her arrival, when she had reluctantly assisted a devout and very sensitive sister named Catherine Warner with laying out procedures. Lily had expected to be afraid of this task: she had not seen a dead person before, and her imagination had run riot – perhaps his ghost would haunt her if she didn't do things right. Men told many tales of ghostly apparitions stalking the battlefields, and back in England quite a few women had sought out spiritualists in the hope of connecting with their dead sweethearts. As she pushed her trolley of soapy water, bandages and tape behind bed screens, however, she was relieved to see a peaceful expression on the dead man's face. Only a few days earlier his weary face had been etched with pain. He was young, only 24, with handsome features and a tall strong build. He had succumbed to a post-operative infection that had raged through his body like a whirlwind. In respectful silence, sister Warner tenderly washed his body as though he could still feel every touch. When they had finished the laying out process they said prayers for the young man's soul. Sister Warner whispered to Lily that it was the last thing on earth they could do for this unfortunate man; she also explained that praying helped her to cope with losing such young patients in tragic circumstances. As the sister completed forms, Lily pushed her trolley slowly back to the sluice and disposed of soiled dressings and unwanted garments before returning to her other duties. For a few days Lily could not shake off the image or memory of the young male corpse. Cynthia, Bessie, Emma and Daisy (a new recruit) were supportive as usual. Not for the first time, Lily wondered how on earth she would cope without her friends. Dora too had spent some time consoling Lily. In the coming days Lily kept all British men in her daily prayers: it was the least she could do.

Above the hustle and bustle of everyday hospital routines, nurses did find time to pray and were, for the most part, devout believers in God. Their Christian ethos underpinned all their activities. For instance, ward sisters would lead all of their staff in prayers at the start and finish of each day. Nurses were continually reminded not to judge patients, staff or visitors. Forgiveness, devout service and self-sacrifice were stressed as the key attributes of a good nurse. There were times when faith was sorely tested, however, and Lily could never quite bring herself to pray for the enemy, although she knew well enough that Jesus had preached that people should love their enemies. She was also quite convinced that the Good Lord might make an exception if he could see the terrible injuries being inflicted on Allied soldiers. But during one of their leisurely walks, Dora firmly corrected her on this point: the Lord did not make any exceptions; everyone was supposed to love one another. An indignant Lily refused to budge from her viewpoint, so eventually they agreed to differ.

Across the green lawns with their budding shrubbery, Colonel Clark mulled over his paperwork. He was fuming. A recent letter from the War Office had informed him that the government would no longer pay for drugs or dressings. He had been given no time to make contingency plans. Writing a first draft of a complaint letter, he penned, 'How did they think he could run a hospital without vital supplies? What was he supposed to do? Conjure them up from thin air?' He stopped for a moment, picked up his first draft, crumpled the paper and threw it into the bin. He did not want to come across as a ranting out of control commanding officer. Perhaps he should gather his thoughts for a while. He got out of his somewhat rickety chair, strolled along the corridor and ordered some tea. Following a short break and a brisk stroll around the grounds, he returned to his desk and penned a letter to the Assistant Director of Medical Services (ADMS) in France to complain about the War Office's decision. Reading between the lines, his anger was thinly disguised. He was further incensed by another War Office letter which asked him to expand the number of hospital beds. Spring and summer, he was informed, heralded a time for new Allied military offensives, and more beds would be needed to cope with increased casualty numbers.

Feeling slightly refreshed after his tea and walk, Colonel Clark attacked his paperwork with renewed vigour. Along with a curt letter to the War Office, a complaint letter to ADMS, he also wrote letters to the War Committee of the Order, Lady Ethel Perrott, Lady Superintendent in Chief of the Nursing Divisions and Earl Ranfurly, who was Director of the Ambulance Department of the Order. These letters were to inform them of the new situation and ask for further funding to buy necessary dressings and drugs for the patients. Clark had made some brief enquiries and discovered that he could save at least £150 a month by purchasing dressings locally.

Having confronted the drugs and dressings problem, Clark turned his attention to other matters. He needed to appoint a new chef, as there were problems with the current chef's timekeeping and cooking standards. The quartermaster was having problems balancing the hospital's accounts, apparently because local tradesmen were not very good at presenting their bills at appropriate times. Tea leaves were still blocking up drains, despite bold notices which forbade orderlies from emptying teapot contents down drains. He also had a visit from the new assistant matron, Sister Templeton, who was complaining about Matron's new rotation scheme for sisters. Chitty had left the hospital before Christmas in order to care for her ailing mother back in England. Sister Templeton was appointed as the new assistant matron on 10 December 1915. Clearly there was some ongoing tension between the matron and her assistant, but Clark had other, more important things to deal with. In order to acquiesce to War Office requests he had to find space for another 220 beds. This was not an easy task. He shelved his existing plans for new officers' rooms and new nurses' cubicles, much to the disappointment of all concerned. He redrew some ward boundaries and walls and then included areas where cubicles were originally to be built. He took these new plans to the quartermaster, who organised construction parties to implement them with due haste.

In addition to planning ward extensions, Clark also had to deal with injured and sick members of staff. His weekly report dated 23 March 1916 stated:

I regret to say that the following casualties have occurred since I last wrote:

Captain Callum our anaesthetist while watching some soldiers at bomb practice was hit in the back by an exploding bomb. A piece of shell entered his back and was extracted by Maynard Smith the same afternoon, he has progressed favourably from the first and will soon be about again. The injury is not likely to cause after effects.

Sergeant Curr, in charge of the sanitary squad, was seized with a stroke and lies here in this hospital in a serious condition. He is a young man of thirty five years of age, of sober and steady habits; and such an attack is unusual under the circumstances and the exact cause has not been arrived at.

Private Hare, Mess waiter has contracted a mild attack of measles or German measles and has been taken to the isolation hospital here.

By the end of March, ward extensions were well under way, and in preparation for large casualty figures, Clark wrote out a new order of instructions for incoming wounded as follows:

Arrangements made for convoy of incoming wounded (on receipt of notice)

1 Refer to book to see whether A. or B. team are on duty.
2 Warn messenger to be at railway siding half an hour before ambulance train is stated to arrive.
3 Advise N.C.O.s of party concerned to warn their men to hold themselves in readiness for the time stated.
4 N.C.O. in charge of unloading must take his men to get out necessary stretchers and blankets (not less than 16 and not more than 48) fifteen minutes before train is due.
5 See that reception room is fully prepared fifteen minutes before train is due – Senior Clerk must see that all necessary note paper etc., is on tables.
6 The night N.C.O. is responsible that the boiler fire and other stoves are in order.
7 The small reception room is only required when there are more than thirty sitting cases.

He also wrote out careful guidelines for staff involved with taking patients to the operating theatre:

When an operation is to take place in the operating theatre the sister of the theatre will see that the case is in theatre ten minutes before advertised time. The General Duty Orderly (G.D.O.) detailed for the purpose will go to the ward or wards and bring the patients.

The sister of the ward will send the ward orderly with the patient to assist with the trolley. The orderly will then return immediately to his ward. The sister of the ward will send with the patient to the theatre his head board, and towel.

The G.D.O. will remain at the disposal of the Theatre sister
until completion of the operation.

With some satisfaction, Colonel Clark put down his pen.
Everything was in order and his guidelines clear and concise.
He was not to know that casualties would soon arrive thick and
fast without warning; a tumbling tidal wave of mutilated bodies,
each and every one of them would need multiple operations.
There would be no time to read instructions.

7

Early summer in Northern France was a joy to behold. Hillsides were brimming with yellow vetch, gorse bushes, buttercups and celandines. Fields of vibrant red poppies adorned the landscape, and clutches of white and purple wild violets circled tree trunks. A proliferation of ox-eye daisies bordered roads and hedgerows, interspersed with tall grasses. Each day before the trumpeted reveille, Lily, who was now working a spell of night duty, took her chair outside on to a covered pathway to enjoy an unofficial tea break. Depending on her workload, this quiet sojourn took place sometime between 4 and 5 a.m. and lasted about fifteen to twenty minutes. Occasionally she would even find time to make toast to accompany her tea. Lily cherished this time; she would listen to the dawn chorus, a cacophony of birdsong that cheerfully broke through the silence, and watch the changing skyline as night turned to day. It seemed to Lily as though these early mornings were cocooned from reality, there was no rumble of distant guns, no circling of reconnaissance aeroplanes, just simple tranquillity: it was a small oasis of peace.

Lily began her stint of night duty on a surgical ward but was later moved to an officers' ward to replace a VAD who had succumbed to a fever. Nurses nicknamed officers' wards 'brass hat' wards. They, along with medical staff and orderlies, also began to refer to the Brigade Hospital simply as 'St John's'. Nicknames were usually coined in an affectionate manner, shortened versions of names or a play on spellings. Étaples was known as 'Eat Apples' for example, and Ypres as 'Wipers'. Friendly banter between men cemented camaraderie and increased levels of empathy. However, there were a few instances recorded where men were singularly unsympathetic to shell shock sufferers.

In terms of administering medical care, military commanders considered it best to maintain a strict hierarchy. Officers, they argued, would not want to appear vulnerable or sick in front of their men, and similarly, other ranks would be reluctant to exhibit any trace of weakness in front of their leaders. In Lily's experience, officers seemed to be quite stoical, unselfish individuals, often asking her if she could find out snippets of information about the wellbeing of their men. Undoubtedly, officers were able to obtain a few luxuries and were treated more leniently than other ranks, but they were still expected to adhere to certain guidelines, and these were updated on a daily basis. Indeed, if wards were quiet then nursing staff would be expected to copy out lists of current guidelines in preparation for pinning on noticeboards. In addition to rules which outlined codes of general behaviour, guidelines included safety information relating to current health problems. For example, officers were warned not to buy fruit from local fruit sellers, primarily because their produce was grown in dirty conditions and washed in dirty water. Dirty fruit was proven to be responsible for several outbreaks of diarrhoea. Additionally, a number of precautions were listed to minimise the spread of epidemics such as mumps, measles, rubella and tuberculosis. Officers were also advised not to frequent certain cafés and brothels where prostitutes were known to have venereal disease. When asked to do so, Lily would carefully copy down these lists of health recommendations, but she often wondered whether any of them would actually be followed.

As Lily finished her night shift, wearily shuffling along the corridors and across the neatly trimmed lawns towards her bed, Matron Todd was beginning her day shift. Minor niggles and tensions between herself and Sister Templeton had irked her recently, particularly since her previous deputy, Mabel Chittock, had such an amiable personality. Included in her early morning prayers, therefore, was a fervent hope that Chitty would soon return and alleviate her from her present incumbent. Undoubtedly there were signs of a personality clash, but much of the tension that existed between Matron and Sister Templeton had arisen because of political differences with regard to the direction and status of nursing. Undoubtedly, nursing politics were fragmented at this stage in professional development. Concern with nurse status was motivated by a desire to escape the dubious 'Mrs Gamp' image* and to provide adequate safeguards for patients. The general consensus of nursing opinion recognised the need for professional status but failed to agree on how best to achieve this goal. They were not sure whether to base their status on social class, religious martyrdom, domestic servitude or military authority. Politically, nurses divided into two camps: those who followed the Florence Nightingale line argued that status rested on the elite standing of the training hospital, while others, led by a Mrs Bedford Fenwick, pressed for state recognition by means of nurse registration. Nightingale had placed great emphasis on the generalist aspect of nursing practice, whereas Bedford Fenwick advocated the need for specialism. Matron Todd's policy of shifting nurses around the hospital in order for them to gain wider experience clearly reflected her bias towards Nightingale's views. Sister Templeton, however, had adopted Fenwick's ideas and vigorously opposed Matron's policy. Professional organisation was in its infancy. The Royal College of Nursing†, established by Conservative politician Sir Arthur Stanley in 1916, initially reflected the views of Nightingale supporters; while the Royal British Nurses Association adopted the policies of Fenwick. Eventually, as College policy shifted direction, both groups pursued the goal

---

* Mrs Gamp was a character created by Charles Dickens and portrayed nurses as gin-soaked women with little if any nursing skill.

† By 1916 there were numerous nursing organisations, but the Royal College of Nursing, established by Sir Arthur Stanley, became the largest and most influential.

of nurse registration. Significantly, this drive towards nurse registration was closely associated with the suffrage movement. War nursing in particular gave added impetus to claims for citizenship, and within the corridors of St John's, nursing sisters gradually became more politicised.

On this early summer morning, however, Matron had other, more pressing considerations on her mind. All senior personnel had been warned of an imminent summer offensive. In preparation for such an event, Matron had drawn up a series of lecture plans, both practical and theoretical. A few of these were basic, such as how to quickly assemble a metal hospital bed frame (usually referred to as cots) in an emergency. Refresher courses in first aid were introduced, which included guidelines as to how to detect severe injuries from those of a minor nature. Often, as Matron pointed out, it was the quiet soldiers who needed more attention rather than those who were able to make considerable noise.

Medical and nursing staff were also instructed on how to use a new innovation in the treatment of orthopaedic conditions – the Thomas splint. Between 1914 and 1916 compound fractures (i.e. fractures that broke through the skin) of the femur were common and lethal. Approximately 80 per cent of all soldiers who sustained this injury died. The Thomas splint was originally designed by Hugh Owen Thomas for treating tuberculosis patients. His nephew, surgeon Robert Jones, however, introduced the splint to the Western front, and another eminent surgeon, Colonel Henry Gray, advocated its widespread use. Prior to this, compound fractures of the femur were simply supported with a pole, rifle, broom handle or anything else that could be rigidly tied to the thigh bone in an attempt to stabilise the fracture. Most soldiers with this injury died of shock before they even reached casualty clearing stations in the field. Bone ends would simply rub together causing extreme shock and heavy blood loss. Often their legs were brutally amputated with kit knives on the battlefield by fellow soldiers attempting to save their lives. With the Thomas splint, femur fractures were aligned and supported by a system of traction and cords, which immobilised the limb and prevented massive blood loss. Subsequently, applications of Thomas splints reduced mortality rates from compound fractures of the femur from 80 per cent to just over 15 per cent. All medical and nursing personnel were eventually taught how to apply and care for patients being treated by the revolutionary new splint. Such patients were usually kept in a base hospital for a period of six weeks, or until an X-ray confirmed that their fractures were healing and no longer labile.

Matron's lecture programme, which began in May, continued until 1 July. Fortunately, she was able to delegate some of the teaching to her senior nursing sisters, and she even persuaded a few medical officers to impart their knowledge to small groups of nurses in their off-duty periods. Medical officers of all base hospitals belonged to medical societies, which enabled them to exchange medical information and research findings. In addition to discussing innovations in wound therapy, infection control, treatments for gas victims and advances in medical technology, health promotion was also considered a priority. Massaging feet with whale oil, for instance, prevented trench foot, as did the frequent changing of socks, and rubbing gums with salt was thought to prevent tooth decay. Yet these simple health promotion measures were not easy for soldiers to adopt on a daily basis. Even senior surgeons had problems in this respect. Dr Harvey Cushing confided to his journal:

> We can manage to circumvent the rats and the imperfect drainage and the dark tents; but we can't keep ahead of the holes in our socks. Roger says that he favours a purse string suture and subsequent trimming with curved scissors borrowed from the operating room. Malcolm we find has been secretly making use of his secretaries, but this is a privilege reserved only for padres. The British War Office should send over a battalion of suffragettes and penalise them

with this task, inscribing on their 'Votes for Women' banners something like: 'Dam the Votes, Darn the Socks'.

Despite inherent failings within health promotion policies, records reveal that most nurses found these new lectures interesting and informative. VADs in particular, who had only received very basic training, acquired considerable knowledge through Matron's lecture programme. However, they were frequently expected to attend lectures in their off-duty time. Orderlies were also invited to learn in this way, but their attendance was sporadic. Lily's close friends, Emma, Bessie, Cynthia and Daisy, organised their own unofficial rota in terms of acquiring knowledge. Each attended a number of lectures but not all, studiously copying down notes for their absent friends. In this way all lecture material was documented and shared appropriately with a minimum of effort.

Whilst Matron was urgently preparing her nurses for an expected avalanche of injured soldiers, Colonel Clark was busy complying with War Office demands to expand bed numbers. Simultaneously he prepared his hospital as far as he was able for the onslaught that would surely follow. He wrote new schedules and procedure notices such as the following evacuation notice:

Sisters in charge of wards will collect and send up to the Registrar's office the medical history sheets of all patients evacuated, immediately they leave their respective wards by night as well as by day.

For example; if an evacuation occurs at 2am the medical history sheets of the patients evacuated should be collected in each ward respectively and sent up to the office at once.

Medical officers should sign the sheets when they mark up the patients for evacuation.

Amidst the ever-increasing number of orders, instructions and procedural guidelines, there were other signs that St John's was preparing for a major influx of battle casualties. The quartermaster began stockpiling dressings and lotions. Larger quantities of food were ordered. Staff vacations were suspended. Orderlies were discreetly digging shallow ditches and creating piles of sandbags in safety precautions that were deliberately kept low key for fear of frightening the nursing staff.

Meanwhile, back in England, Lady Ethel Perrott was responding to Colonel Clark's urgent request for more funding. As Lady Superintendent in Chief, married to the Secretary General of the Order Colonel Sir Herbert Perrott, she was well suited to the task. She was an elegant-looking woman, almost fragile in appearance, with small facial features, high cheekbones, inquisitive eyes and a slender aristocratic nose. Yet appearances in this case were deceptive: Lady Perrott was anything but fragile. Not only did she manage to raise enough funds to keep St John's in perfect working order throughout the war, she also raised enough money to build a hospital chapel. Donations were obtained from a wide variety of sources, and wards were usually named after the most generous fund-raisers. Money poured in from the British War Relief Organisation of America, the Irish War Hospital, Rhode Island relief Society, Newfoundland and New South Wales to name but a few. Lady Perrott was assisted in her fund-raising efforts by senior members of the Order and upper-class philanthropists such as the Duchess of Bedford. The latter had been particularly instrumental in helping to raise the hospital chapel money, which in total cost £372 9s 9d. Attached to the dining hall, the chapel could hold up to 200 people, and it was delicately decorated by a woven altar cloth depicting several crosses of St John.

Lady Perrott did not restrict her efforts to fund-raising. Although Dame Maud McCarthy was in charge of all Allied nurses and members of the Queen Alexandra's Imperial Military Nursing Service (QAIMNS), Lady Perrott was superintendent of the Order of St John nurses. Working tirelessly behind the scenes, she was responsible for recruitment, vetting and deployment of suitable nurses. She also maintained a close working relationship with the commanding officer and Matron Todd, and made several visits to the Brigade Hospital to ensure that funds were spent in an appropriate manner. Intelligent, astute and fiercely determined, Lady Perrott was the driving force behind hospital fund-raising and organisation. Moreover, these crucial fund-raising activities sustained the Brigade Hospital throughout the entire war.

8

By June 1916 the area around Étaples was home to about 100,000 British and Commonwealth troops. Billeted in surrounding houses or camped out in large tents, they were put through their paces on a daily basis by enthusiastic sergeant majors. Feeling confident, these troops were eager to put their trench warfare skills into practice. Most of the British troops preparing for battle consisted of volunteers who belonged to 'pals brigades', men who had joined up together in large groups. They were friends who had enlisted from the same village, community or work place. With a strong sense of camaraderie and a good deal of optimism, they were convinced that the Germans would soon capitulate under the weight of a new British advance.

As base hospitals in France geared up for the summer offensive, General Arthur Sloggett, Director General of the Army Medical Services in the Field and a Knight of Grace of the Order of St John, drew up contingency medical plans on a much wider scale. Sloggett had joined the army as a surgeon in 1881 and was one of the most experienced officers within the RAMC. A tall, trim gentleman with poker-straight posture, he had thick white, receding hair, a neatly trimmed white moustache, deep chiselled features and a firm-set jawline. His bravery in the field had earned him a plethora of awards and medals, and he was held in high esteem by the men he commanded. Furthermore, preparing medical arrangements for fighting men was second nature to him. With meticulous precision, his plans for the medical care of battle casualties reflected a high degree of thoroughness and efficiency.

In preparation for the Somme offensive, field ambulances were divided into two sections, one placed very near to the front line and the other slightly behind. It was anticipated that these sections would rapidly amalgamate if necessary, thus providing large, advanced casualty clearance dressing stations. Specialist medical teams, which included anaesthetists, and orthopaedic and neurological surgeons, were placed on call; makeshift operating theatres were moved to forward areas. In addition, three fully equipped hospital trains were placed on standby in order to transport seriously wounded men from casualty clearance stations to base hospitals. Sloggett had also ensured that further hospital trains were available if necessary. He had no reason to doubt the efficacy of his plans. Indeed, his medical arrangements worked extremely well in theory; they turned out, however, to be woefully inadequate in practice. In fairness to Sloggett, he had ensured that more numbers of medical personnel were on the front line than during previous battles. Moreover, it was highly unlikely that anyone could have predicted the scale of carnage engendered by the Somme offensive. On the contrary, senior military officers and their men were reasonably confident of a successful attack with only light casualties.

Officially intended as a combined French and British attack, the main Allied Somme offensive of 1916 became a predominantly British battle. Instigated along a 30km line, which ran from the northern section of the River Somme, the battle was preceded by heavy artillery bombardment of German positions. This bombardment lasted for eight days and was thought to have considerably weakened German defences. At 7.30 a.m. on 1 July the Battle of the Somme began; within an hour and a half, 20,000 British soldiers had been killed. By the end of the day there were nearly 60,000 British casualties. The German soldiers had simply taken shelter in deep concrete dugouts during the waves of artillery fire and emerged to machine gun British troops as they walked slowly towards them. A young soldier who took part in the offensive, named Private W. Roberts, wrote in his diary:

Opened a violent bombardment on the German lines 7am and 7.30 advance started. We were the 4th Battalion to go over, which we did about an hour later. The short but terrible rush through the fierce curtain fire with men falling on all sides I shall never forget. High explosive shells fell all around us. The sights I saw are too terrible to write about and men almost blown to pieces were lying side by side. Unable to proceed further, the order to retire was given and I thanked God that I came through the terrible ordeal unhurt. I went to work in our frontline at night but had to come away as it was almost blown to pieces. There again I saw dead and wounded lying side by side. Some were moaning and others had so far lost their reason that they were laughing and singing. July 2nd. Resting in one of the trenches but went to carry wounded out at 11. The communication trench out, was packed with stretchers. Tear shells were sent over which burst about the entrance of our trenches and my eyes were running with water. Returned to our resting trench about day break. July 3rd. On sentry duty in the battered front line, dead men, rifles spades and equipment were lying about and there I had to stay till 2am next morning.[*]

Other reports were similar. John Buchan, who produced a pamphlet entitled 'The Battle of the Somme 1916', recorded:

The British moved forward in line after line, dressed as if on parade; not a man wavered or broke ranks; but minute by minute the ordered lines melted away under the deluge of high explosives, shrapnel, rifle and machine gun fire. The splendid troops shed their blood like water for the liberty of the world.

---

[*]   Transcript of the diary of Private W. Roberts July 1916. Durham Record Office ref: D/DLI 7/577/2.

Walking slowly towards the enemy had proved to be a disaster, and since officers led the attack, they were more likely to have been killed or severely injured. Sixty per cent of all officers who took part in the first day of the Somme battle were killed. The men who followed them into battle were simply mown down by enemy fire at a phenomenal rate. One eyewitness claimed that men went down at such speed he thought someone had given them an order to lie down.

Casualty clearance stations were soon overwhelmed. A basic triage system assessed the injured upon arrival, and many men were simply placed to one side and left to die; others, unable to access medical assistance, died where they fell. Those who were fortunate enough to reach first-aid posts and advanced dressing stations were quickly treated with rudimentary dressings. As many of the injured as possible were placed on hospital trains and shipped back to England. Casualty numbers were so high that only the most seriously wounded could be kept in France. By 3 p.m. on 1 July news of the appallingly high casualty figures gradually filtered through to Sloggett, and he called the rail transport office at Amiens to urgently order more hospital trains. Some of these, however, took over ten hours to reach the Somme. By this time base hospitals were also overrun with wounded. Every conceivable mode of transport had been commandeered to shift wounded men away from the battlefield towards some semblance of care, and medical personnel worked around the clock to help the injured. Walking wounded were forced to wait for hours in lengthy queues whilst medical officers dealt with massive influxes of stretcher cases.

Base hospitals had sent small parties of nursing sisters down the line to help at dressing stations. Those who remained were instructed to cancel all off-duty periods and wake all nurses who might be slumbering after night duty. With shouts of 'all hands to the pump', sisters promptly gave rapid, abrupt orders to their colleagues as severely injured soldiers were squeezed endlessly through hospital doors. Almost all of these soldiers were labelled with a bright red stripe, which indicated that they might haemorrhage at any moment. Some had been inoculated against tetanus in the field, and these were marked with a 'T' on their forehead. Field cards had been hastily written and attached to uniforms of the wounded. Operating theatres were in full swing and additional operating tables were brought in to cope with excessive demands. St John's hospital had evacuated as many men as possible before the Somme battle commenced, but there were still not enough beds to cope with the numbers of injured. They lay in corridors, in doorways, in recreation rooms and in dining halls; some were even strewn across dining tables or lay on office floors. They stood outside, lined up along duckboards and on verandas, and they were packed like sardines across the lawn so not a bit of grass could be seen.

Official war diary records state that, between the 1 and 5 July 1916, St John Ambulance Brigade Hospital admitted 1,400 soldiers. During these few days, convoys of wounded were brought in mainly by ambulance train. On the 1 July No. 19 ambulance train arrived; on the 2 July No. 11 ambulance train brought in more wounded. On 3 July casualties arrived from the front without warning by road, and on 4 and 5 July ambulance trains numbered 27 and 31 also brought large numbers of injured to the hospital doors. Between them, base hospitals had the capacity to admit 22,000 wounded at any one time. Hospital trains and ships operated a shuttle service but were equally swamped by casualties. During the course of five days, nearly 40,000 injured men were transported to base hospitals in France or to military hospitals in England.

At St John's hospital medical staff quickly managed to establish some order from the ensuing chaos. Surgeons Major Maynard Smith and Captain Hope boomed orders to their theatre staff. Radiographers frantically struggled to X-ray large numbers of men in preparation for treatment. There were piles upon piles of exhausted men, covering every inch of available hospital space. Here the severely injured lay, in excruciating pain, hovering between life and death – some praying for the latter. Their bodies viciously mutilated, blasted apart by relentless artillery and machine gun fire, their uniforms in shreds, their limbs blown away or shattered to pieces, they gazed at nurses with soulless, desolate eyes.

Amidst an ever extending carpet of blood and khaki, nursing sisters, VADs and orderlies attended to their vast array of patients. The place resembled a living hell. Lily had been woken from her slumber at 4 p.m., and henceforth there seemed to be no distinction between night duty and day duty. Everyone just worked to the point of exhaustion. Amongst a pile of seething, groaning bodies Lily noticed a white-faced youth holding on to his side; his eyes were glazing over, and she rushed over to him. His pulse was barely palpable and the right side of his abdomen was blown clean away, blood soaking what remained of his uniform jacket. Lily took a deep breath; she was frightened beyond words. His wounds had exposed muscles that she had only seen in anatomy books. Then the operating theatre door opened suddenly. Lily looked imploringly at the gowned surgeon, quickly telling him that despite his heavy blood loss, the man still had a pulse. He grimly nodded in her direction and beckoned to two orderlies. Between them they managed to get the youth on to a trolley and into theatre. Lily had no time to contemplate his fate. A frantic Emma was trying to stem a haemorrhage from a vicious-looking arm wound, tightening a tourniquet with all the strength she could muster. Bessie had responded to Matron's call for more towels and flannels, not to wash the men but to pack into their abdominal wounds to soak up, and possibly stem, the flow of blood. Cynthia, meanwhile, was giving a cigarette to a man who was evidently dying, while simultaneously wielding a pair of forceps, trying to pick out remnants of a man's uniform from his wound. It was difficult to know which way to turn or who to help first. There were men with half of their faces blown away, some without mouths or chins, but there was no time to express pity or sympathy, or to mourn the departure of those who did not pull through.

Matron was a tower of strength, moving about the hospital floors and grounds with a calm and encouraging manner. Sisters, too, appeared to possess an abundance of calm. Even when faced with the most appalling of injuries and the most trying of circumstances, they remained resolutely serene. Sister Jane Bemrose, efficient and brusque in manner, was particularly good at ushering people around and dishing out clear, concise orders. Sister Margaret Ballance was adept at cajoling people and getting them organised. Sister Dora Little, concerned by the combination of summer heat and large intakes of patients, quietly persuaded senior orderlies to urgently review their sanitary arrangements. Swarms of flies buzzed furiously above open wounds, occasionally settling on exposed, decaying flesh. A pungent smell of disinfectant combined with stale blood permeated the balmy summer air. Rising July temperatures undoubtedly increased the risk of cross infection, but they were welcomed by hundreds of wounded lying in hospital grounds awaiting treatment and also by those who were still stranded on blood-splattered battlefields, abandoned where they had fallen.

Over the next few days, the sight of sisters and nurses kneeling beside their patients on lawns, in corridors and other unlikely locations became commonplace. A few, who had been rudely awakened from sleep, were still adorned in white dressing gowns and slippers. They kept going by sheer force of will, bandaging limbs as fast as was humanly possible and efficiently attending to severe wounds. They cheered the despairing and comforted the dying. Colonel Carr, Deputy Director of Medical Services, visited St John's on 7 July. He spoke to some of the patients and praised staff for their splendid work. On 8 July the hospital water supply failed. The pump had simply worn out under the strain of endlessly supplying water during the previous week. Water was hastily ferried across from other hospitals in the region, and the pump was repaired the following day.

By this stage St John's had expanded by another sixty-four beds, making a total of 740 beds. Other temporary beds were erected for emergency use, but these were not counted as regular beds. Another water filter was brought in to distil water from the chalky soil, and further equipment was bought for the operating theatre. Official surgical reports claimed that:

> Men were in a very collapsed condition following amputations or the opening up of severe gas infection of limbs or body. Ultimate recovery was due mainly to intravenous injection of 2, 3 or at times 4 pints of normal saline solution or 4% sodium bicarbonate, given before leaving the operating theatre.
>
> Blood transfusion was used successfully and there was no untoward result of any kind following blood transfusion.

Furthermore, as Matron frequently pointed out to her staff, the vast majority of these wounded men were young and fit before they were wounded. This fact alone undoubtedly aided recovery in the long term, and many men survived who clearly would not have done so if they had been older or weaker.

Matron did her very best to lift staff morale during this difficult time. She offered a listening ear, a kindly word and, when all else failed, a carefully measured 4oz tot of brandy. For the most part, her nursing sisters and VADs were genteel Edwardian ladies, more accustomed to elegant study rooms, libraries and drawing rooms than to the blood and guts of conflict. Before their arrival in France, some may have conjured up romantic images of nursing, mopping a fevered brow or gently reading to a handsome, heroic patient. Stark reality bore no relation to romantic preconceptions. Indeed, for those who harboured them, the Battle of the Somme was a baptism of fire. Moreover, even nurses who were more realistic could not have conceived carnage on such a grand scale. Yet without exception nurses coped, tending the wounded relentlessly, working flat out, skipping meals and rest periods until they were almost dead on their feet.

However, the strain of nursing under such stressful conditions took its toll. Sister Little succumbed to a fever, Sister Margaret Ballance was charged with so much adrenaline that she was unable to sleep and Sister Warner suffered with blisters and swollen ankles. Lily complained of throbbing headaches, whereas Emma repeatedly convinced herself that she had forgotten something important, some piece of medical information that perhaps she had failed to pass on to medical officers in charge; this feeling continually haunted her and prevented her from resting adequately. Bessie had bandaged so many limbs that her fingers were red raw and her hands swollen. Daisy, who was the most petite and fragile looking of all the nurses, claimed one morning that her feet were so swollen she could not possibly go on duty. Ten minutes later, however, she donned her uniform, wincing with pain as she reluctantly forced her feet into her little black boots. Cynthia, meanwhile, almost crying with tiredness, fought back her tears on a daily basis, stoically refusing to succumb to exhaustion. She would start her day by praying, washing, eating and more praying. Then she dragged her uniform on, grabbed a clean apron and pushed her cap firmly on to her head. She couldn't give in. Every nurse was needed every single day and through the night-time too: patients were overflowing, tasks numerous, suffering immense and grief overwhelming. Yet despite her efforts, Cynthia collapsed on 12 July and was ordered to stay in bed for at least three days. Other nurses would follow suit.

9

On 14 July 1916 Colonel James Clark relinquished his position as hospital commanding officer in order to return to England, where he resumed his previous post as Chief Commissioner of the Brigade. He had been agitating to leave for some time, because his original remit was to establish the hospital and to get it running in an efficient manner. He had succeeded in this task and was now eager to get home to his family. He handed over command of the hospital to Major Charles Trimble, who was later promoted to colonel. In normal circumstances this occasion would have been marked by a big farewell party, but this was impossible when hospital staff were under such strain. Clark's departure was, therefore, a very low-key affair. A few senior officers gathered in the officers' mess to thank him for his services and toast his future; then it was on with the job, with no time for sentiment. Prior to the Somme offensive, patient intakes were a mixture of sitting and walking wounded, along with a few stretcher cases. Now nearly all patients were brought in on stretchers and most arrived without warning. Some of these patients had not even seen a casualty clearing station, as Trimble noted in one of his weekly reports to Lord Ranfurly back at St John's Gate in London. Dated 19 July 1916, this report stated:

> On the 15th we received a convoy of ninety five wounded, the condition of these men was certainly exceedingly bad, they came down directly from the fighting line and their wounds were of a most serious nature. This has kept the surgical division of the hospital very busy.

Yet despite the strain these casualties placed on the hospital, Trimble's later report of 27 July is reassuring:

> A very large proportion of cases were received on stretchers and the number of badly wounded vary considerably. I think it is customary to send this hospital seriously wounded cases and it is particularly justifiable as we are in every way capable of dealing with them.

In addition to injured soldiers, many stretcher-bearers were wounded or killed. Over 400 RAMC orderlies were killed in the Somme offensive alone. They risked their lives on a daily basis as they struggled to rescue mangled men from theatres of conflict. They too were working under extreme duress, trying to retrieve the injured while relentless enemy fire bore down on them. They could not reach everyone. Hundreds of wounded died where they had fallen; others waited days to be discovered.

An officer from the East Lancashire Regiment was admitted eight days after the start of the battle. He had lain in a shell crater next to three corpses until a stretcher-bearer finally found him, severely dehydrated, with a foul-smelling soporific leg wound. Exhausted, vomiting intermittently, ears humming and eyes watering, he had lost all sense of time. He had managed to crawl over to one side of the crater and drink some water from the water bottles of his dead comrades, and he had also eaten small amounts of bully beef. He remembered shouting loudly for help, particularly at nightfall, because he thought it would be safer for someone to rescue him under cover of darkness, but no one had heard his cries. Confused and barely conscious upon arrival at hospital, his leg was amputated and he responded well to intravenous normal saline. Like many officers, however, his first concern was for his men. Desperate to know how they had fared in battle, he continually asked his nurses for as much information as possible. News, when it came, was almost unbearable. Out of 700 officers and men of the 1st Battalion who went into action, only 237 were able to answer the roll call at the end of the day. Out of 720 men of the 11th Battalion who took part in the attack, 594 were killed or wounded. When informed of the total number of casualties, the officer felt sick to the pit of his stomach. The 11th East Lancashire included the Accrington Pals, vibrant young men who had joined up together, trained together and died together.* Whole villages of men had been wiped out during the first day of the Battle of the Somme, forcing the War Office to re-evaluate recruitment policies.

Conscription was introduced in March 1916, but the steady flow of Somme wounded largely consisted of men who had volunteered their services. Henceforth, however, recruitment polices no longer targeted groups of friends or workplace gatherings. Men were conscripted as individuals, and there were very few exemptions.

Understandably, patients' conversations on hospital wards were dominated by their shared battle experiences and feelings of hate towards the enemy. Those who had lain out on battlefields for some length before rescue also described their gruesome surroundings. They recalled evil smells of rotting flesh crawling with maggots as murders of crows circled over the dying and pecked at the dead; faces of dead men, with fixed glassy-eyed stares; odours of fulminating gas gangrene bacillus carried on summer breezes, turning the air toxic; and eerily wraithlike figures, adorned with helmets and scraps of uniform, scattered across blood-flooded fields.

Weighed down by responsibility, brass hat wards were full of officers who were wracked with guilt. Prematurely aged by the accountability of command, they were plagued by images of the men they had led into battle and who had subsequently perished.

---

*   Further information can be obtained from the Lancashire Infantry Museum Fulwood Barracks, Preston, PR2 8AA.

Distressing scenes of tremendous, unprecedented bloodshed tortured their minds. These officers had known their doomed men well: they had censored their letters home and knew intimate details of their home lives. They could list the names of men whose wives had given birth in their absence, those who had sick mothers or fathers and those who were engaged to their sweethearts, looking forward to marriage.

On officers' wards across clusters of base hospitals, haunting spectres of battlefield savagery hung in the air, like ominous clouds refusing to disperse. A pervading despondency had taken hold of these senior military men, one that was impossible to shake off. Lily too was in despondent mood. At times, tiredness combined with feelings of hopelessness threatened to overwhelm her. The youth with abdominal injuries she had earlier attended to died of his wounds on 19 July. Matron was sympathetic and gently explained to Lily that patients with such severe abdominal wounds rarely survived, adding that his death was a blessed relief from suffering. But try as she might, Lily could not see things this way. She could only see the waste and pity of his suffering and demise. She hadn't known the youth, she had only responded to his pain, but there had been something in his plaintive eyes that had resonated with her. She managed to suppress her grief whilst on duty, but she cried softly to herself every night for a week.

Lily was not alone in suppressing her emotions; tempers were frayed, and everyone was tired, emotionally drained and physically debilitated. Even Bessie, who was usually full of the joys of living, had been sombre of late. Emma was quieter than usual, and Daisy looked on the point of collapse. Sisters Dora Little and Jane Bemrose had dark shadows below their eyes, and Sister Ballance looked pale and overwrought. Only Matron seemed to be able to rise above the surroundings. Constantly praising her nurses for their splendid work in the face of adversity, she urged them to smile more in an effort to lift the men's spirits. Matron, who rolled her sleeves up and worked every bit as hard as everyone else, was now described by some of her staff as a professional optimist. Nothing appeared to faze her or put her out of sorts. This was an accurate observation of her character. Constance Todd was naturally very cheerful and practical, firmly believing that hard work was an antidote to many ills. She comforted her patients and nurses with an equal measure of compassion and pragmatism, and her door was open to everyone. Even Sister Templeton, who was often at loggerheads with Matron, was forced to concede that Matron's dignified strength of character was exemplary. She was a rock of impeccable calm in the midst of an ongoing disaster.

Matron herself took solace in faith. Moreover, as a devout Christian, she believed unwaveringly in the power of prayer. She was not immune to the sorrow and suffering that surrounded her; she simply offered her prayers and thoughts to Christ her Saviour. In addition to her most private prayers, she also prayed humbly for the strength to continue her work, for guidance in decision making, and for an end to the bitter conflict which had engulfed the world. After morning prayers, when time permitted she recorded some details of hospital life, writing to her family:

We increased the nursing staff of sisters and V.A.Ds but some of our orderlies were taken away for work up the line. With the exception of one midnight visit from a zeppelin which dropped a number of bombs, none of which exploded, we were very free from alarm.

One day an empty German observation balloon which had somehow got away from the line, drifted over us – the anchor hanging from it carried off part of the roof of the sister's mess; then uprooted a huge telegraph post in front of the hospital bringing it and all the live wires down to the ground, but no one was hurt and the balloon drifted quietly out to sea.

On 28 July Newfoundland's Premier visited St John's to boost the morale of soldiers from the Royal Newfoundland Regiment. They had begun their advance on the Somme at 8.45 a.m. on 1 July and had sustained a 90 per cent casualty rate. Within minutes the whole regiment was virtually wiped out. The hospital's new commanding officer, Charles Trimble, escorted Premier Morris around the hospital, but the men were lethargic, pallid and largely uncommunicative. On the same day, No. 30 ambulance brought in another convoy of men, consisting of sixty-six wounded and fourteen sick. The following day a further seventy-eight wounded and two sick men arrived at St John's. In his official war correspondence, Trimble made a special note on 31 July 1916: 'During recent fighting wounds have been of a very severe nature. Compound fractures of legs and arms with gas infected wounds being numerous; shell fire appears to have accounted for these injuries.'

Infections of gas gangrene posed the biggest problem for surgeons as they frantically tried to save lives. It was a race against time, and amputations were the most common of all base hospital operations. In an effort to prevent the spread of gangrene, around 10 per cent of all amputations were carried out at casualty clearing stations. A few were brutally carried out on the battlefield with nothing more than a sharpened kit knife. Those casualties who managed to access front-line medical care were also given anti-tetanus serum and the typhoid vaccine. Furthermore, the policy of moving qualified medical staff and casualty clearing stations nearer to the front undoubtedly improved casualty survival rates, as did improvements in transport. As Harvey Cushing recalled in his journal:

> In the early days things were badly organized and conditions were shocking. The wounded were all rushed south as rapidly as possible and the more seriously ill were put off whenever or wherever trains stopped. They were picked up in anyway chance may favour – luckily if by ambulance, but more often

than not by a cattle or provision train returning from the front. One of these trains had dumped about five hundred badly wounded men and had left them lying between the tracks in the rain, with no cover whatsoever. One English officer had been six days thus in transport with a musket for a splint tied to a compound fracture of the femur, no dressing whatsoever, almost no food or drink; he was in delirium when he arrived.

Commenting on work in an early casualty clearing station, Cushing noted:

The entire convoy of cases has been sorted over, relabelled and passed on, and the great room is empty except for a few men who need immediate attention; a brachial artery is being tied for a secondary haemorrhage by a junior medical officer. It is all very simple – nothing as elaborate as an x-ray machine and no beds except the few for officers. In one large room, under a new wooden roof – for a Taube dropped a bomb on the old one ten days ago – there were closely packed rows of wounded awaiting further transport, lying on their stretchers with their muddy boots protruding from heavy blankets. In one row were seventeen head cases – men in every possible stage of inter-cranial injury. Many of them needing immediate attention.

Men cite their name, regiment, the place he received the injury and under what circumstances, how long he had had his clothes on without changing them and where he got his first, second and possibly third dressing before he reached the ambulance.

Observing several hospital buildings that did not meet the standard of St John's, Cushing stated:

Some are not well built. For business only, unadorned, unattractive, and some day, the heat reflected from the sand dunes onto these corrugated iron buildings will make them nigh on intolerable. Some of the wards were bad – so narrow that one row of cots were placed end on; and the doors wide enough for a stretcher were too narrow to transmit a cot. But criticism is cheap and there was much to commend.

Clearly, medical preparations for the Somme battles, however inadequate they proved to be, were still a great improvement on previous medical arrangements, being more thorough and better organised. Furthermore, in terms of medical equipment, casualty clearing stations were becoming more like small base hospitals. This trend continued throughout the war. However, the position of casualty clearing stations always posed a dilemma for senior military personnel: they needed to be far enough forward to administer care but not too far forward because then they ran the risk of impeding military combat missions.

Wound treatments had also improved, and mortality rates from wound sepsis had more than halved. But as July drew to a close, nursing sisters were more concerned about the wounds that could not be seen, rather than those clearly visible to the naked eye. Of those who had seen action on the Somme, 40 per cent were suffering from shell shock (neurasthenia). This was a dramatic rise compared to previous battles, and officers were just as likely to be affected by the condition as men in other ranks. All of them, in various degrees, were infused with a palpable sense of fear. Some men were frightened of going to sleep because night terrors haunted their dreams, and were scared to eat or wash; others were simply unable to function on any level. One handsome young captain had developed a severe stammer and an uncontrollable muscle spasm. Lily thought it was as though his words were going to describe something so utterly dreadful that he simply couldn't voice them. Another officer was haunted by visions, which repeatedly came without warning into his mind at random moments, of a man he had bayoneted; no matter how hard he tried, this unrelenting image followed him wherever he went.

As officers were more likely to be killed or injured, the hospitals had to accommodate accordingly. According to Matron's letters, St John's expanded the number of officer beds from fifty-six to eighty-eight in order to cope with rising officer casualties. Other base hospitals also expanded their officer bed capacity. Moreover, the growing number of officers displaying symptoms of neurasthenia prompted alarm in military commanders and greater sympathy in medical circles. Nurses found it increasingly distressing to care for neurasthenia victims, since no amount of comforting or compassion could sooth their minds. As Lily confided to Emma after a particularly hard day, it was heart breaking to see so many officers inflicted in such a way, and extremely upsetting. After all, these men were the military elite: they could usually be relied upon in a crisis; were renowned for being upstanding, honourable and principled; were trained in leadership skills; and were at their peak of physical fitness. Lily felt that somehow it was more disturbing to see officers severely shell-shocked than it was to witness men in the ranks with the condition. She was convinced that officers on her brass hat ward had been stripped of their masculinity, reduced to gibbering wrecks or mere shadows of their previous selves.

As the war progressed it became abundantly clear that officers were four times more likely to suffer from neurasthenia than the men they led into battle. However, neurasthenia remained a controversial subject. Dr Charles Meyers, a Cambridge psychologist, had published a paper on the subject as early as 1915. He argued that officers were more likely to suffer from the condition because they were forced to repress their emotions in front of their men. In 1916 he tried to prevent the execution of shell shock sufferers for cowardice and to convince senior army commanders that shell shock could be cured by cognitive therapy. According to Meyers, sufferers needed rest, recuperation, behavioural techniques, relaxation by means of reading or taking up artistic pursuits and, most importantly of all, talking therapies. His tutor, Dr William Rivers, held similar ideas and was responsible for establishing Craiglockhart military psychiatric hospital in 1916. This institution was nicknamed as 'dottyville' by one of its famous residents, war poet Siegfred Sassoon. Eventually, as demand continued to grow, twenty hospitals specialising in neurasthenia treatments were established across Britain.

Nevertheless, this did not reflect an acceptance of neurasthenia within military circles. Indeed, the views of Myers and Rivers were often marginalised in favour of those who treated neurasthenia as an emotional weakness, a disciplinary problem, a failure to recognise a sense of duty or simply an attempt to escape the front line. Canadian-born Lewis Yealland, for instance, boasted that he could return all supposedly shell-shocked victims to the front line in a matter of days. By his own admission, he did not believe that shell shock existed but claimed to have a 100 per cent success rate in terms of 'curing' men of such weakness. He relied on auto-suggestion methods, solitary confinement, aversion therapies and electric shock therapy. He firmly believed that shell shock was merely an insidious form of collective hysteria, and his methods were barbaric. He was renowned, for example, for tying uncommunicative soldiers to chairs, simultaneously applying electric shocks to the back of their tongues and other sensitive areas whilst shouting at them to become heroes. These soldiers were required to speak in order to stop this torture, and some could not do so and were repeatedly subjected to the same treatment.

Yet the suffering of soldiers during the first month of the Somme offensive had highlighted the fact that any one of them could be struck down by neurasthenia. It could not be claimed that officers were weak minded or that they were prone to bouts of hysteria. As Lily and her colleagues had observed, these shell-shocked men were brave, decisive leaders, and many more of their ilk would suffer the same fate in the months to come.

10

As the Somme offensive entered its second month, there was
no let up in the number of casualties that came streaming in
through the doors of St John's. Trimble's weekly report dated
2 August 1916 highlights the continuing strain on hospital staff:

All convoys stretcher cases and wounds very severe.
Compound fractures of thighs arms and G.S.W.s of head
chest and abdomen. Dealing with these cases has entailed
a considerable amount of very heavy work on the part of
surgical and nursing staff.

At the present time the hospital is discharging the duties
of a surgical institution; there have been very few medical
cases, some instances of gas poisoning from shell fumes came
under observation.

A further report dated 16 August 1916 gives some indication
of the continual flow of casualties:

Between the 9th and the 15th we received three convoys
of wounded, one consisted of four special stretcher cases
admitted from No. 15 Ambulance train. These were all of
an exceedingly serious nature and one man died an hour
and a half after admission. The second convoy arrived at
2.15am on the 11th, and numbered thirty two stretcher
and sixty three sitting cases. The third was received on
the 13th at 12.55am and numbered seventy two – all of
which were stretcher cases, and as usual composed of most
dangerously wounded men. We had some trouble at the

pumping station on the 9th and very urgent orders were issued to curtail supply as much as possible. I am glad to say the water was again alright on the following day. I can also report that the hospital now has three thousand socks in store!

For the men who had been struggling to darn their socks, the latter piece of news was most welcome. An urgent appeal for new socks had been sent out to the British public, and they had responded generously to the call. An avalanche of letters also arrived during the middle of August. A new nursing sister named Elsie Goodman was the recipient of most of this correspondence. With curly blonde hair, large deep blue eyes and a pretty, pale, delicate face, Elsie was the object of considerable male attention. One of a group of unseasoned sisters drafted in to strengthen numbers in preparation for the Somme battles, she had arrived in June and was immediately assigned to an officer ward. In July she confided to her diary:

> I am liking it here very much and could never have thought I would for a moment. Of course there will always be days when the horror of nursing it all unnerves one.
>
> I have met some very nice officers.

Elsie was a natural communicator and avid listener. She seemed to take to the officer ward like a duck to water. She coaxed people along effortlessly to get the best out of them in terms of work, and she was universally liked by both patients and staff. Whilst others referred to patients as 'the man in bed 22' or by their medical condition, Elsie always called her patients by name, often prefixing this with 'darling boy'. At the beginning of August she wrote:

> Those who I have got to know best have been Lt Patterson, nice boy with a wounded hand. Then we had three Australian

officers in. I didn't care much at first for them, but liked them very much after.

I think Lt D. McClean I got to know and like the very best. He is 6th Battalion First Divison and had a G.S.W. of elbow. I had quite a good time with him, but of course he was one of the first to go on.

Then G.L. Cavanaugh – he is very good looking in a flirtatious kind of way. Clever too, though like all of them certainly hid it under a rough exterior, in the way of speech etc. He stayed a long time because of his knee. He was in the machine gun corps.

Then there is Captain Tozer A.A.M.C. who had a rather miraculous escape; having had a piece of shrapnel travel right across his brain, and lodge itself in the back. After a few days of being semi-unconscious he gradually became alright, apparently none the worse for wear.

For Lily, whose natural inclination was to be quite shy and awkward around men, Elsie's ease of social interaction with the opposite sex was something to be admired. Indeed, many of the sisters were slightly envious of Elsie, who not only established excellent relationships with her patients during their time at St John's but continued to stay in touch with her 'darling boys' long after they were discharged.

Lily often wondered how on earth Elsie found the time to answer her mountain of letters. Though she herself occasionally received missives from ex-patients, like the following from a Private Davis:

We have just come out of the trenches for a rest, we have had rather a warm time of it. Sorry to say that I have lost my chum and have had many a narrow escape myself, but we are all in the best of spirits fighting for dear England.

I wish I could hear the gramophone, it would be better than bursting shells but never mind; we have our own duty to do, which we are trying our best to do to the last, like many more brave fellows … last week it was miserable out here but it is a little better this week.

Private Davis was killed in action two weeks after sending this letter. Lily also received a letter from one of her nursing friends back in England, informing her of the death of another ex-patient:

> With regard to Lt. Corporal R Mason, First Black Watch. As you know … Mason went to France with the first B.E.F., was wounded in the Battle of Mons. He returned to France and was wounded again in December 1915. After being in hospital for some months he was recommended for the D.C.M. for bringing in three wounded men under fire. But he was in the big push in July 1916 and lost his life with five others by a shell exploding.
>
> There have been difficult days, but these are utterly insignificant compared with the joys of success; of seeing sick men get well, sad ones made happy, all possible through the splendid work of our keen, capable and unselfish staff. All honour to them! Their record is fine and we hope to continue with the same enthusiasm and fine esprit de corps.

Such letters always filled Lily with sorrow and a sense of humility. At times she was very downhearted, but she forced a smile for her patients nonetheless. Often she felt as though she were an actress, stepping into character the moment she donned her uniform.

It was 15 August, and the day began much like any other. All wards were heavy and busy; but Lily had a half-day off and had made plans to meet other staff members in Paris Plage for afternoon tea. Once her shift was finished she changed into a cool white blouse and long black skirt. Placing her uniform straw hat firmly on her head, she cycled slowly to her destination in the sticky, oppressive summer heat. There, as she propped up her rickety bicycle against an ancient-looking white stone wall, she heard a man shouting for help. Turning sharply around, she caught a faint glimpse of Captain McCloy from the pathology laboratory being taken rapidly out to sea on the ebbing tide. He was waving his arms frantically, his silhouette diminishing in size by the second. Recognising that McCloy was in terrible danger, Lieutenant Coe (later a captain), the dental surgeon, swam vigorously out to save him. However, the undercurrent was so strong that he too got into trouble. Luckily the quartermaster, Lieutenant Hine, was also at hand and dived in to rescue both men. An immense struggle ensued as Hine and Coe battled strenuously against the tide and enormous waves to bring Captain McCloy back to safety. By this time the dramatic situation had attracted quite an audience. Lily managed to acquire a few warm, woollen blankets from some local women and organised some piping hot drinks. Hine and Coe received a hearty round of applause as they reached the shoreline, along with plenty of praise and attention.* Captain McCloy made a full recovery.

Lily could not settle in the tea shop for long, so decided to go for a short walk along the beach before returning to Étaples. It had not turned out to be a relaxing afternoon off, but at least she had an exciting story to tell her friends on her return. Beginning her tale along the lines of 'You'll never guess what happened today', Lily recounted the drama of Captain McCloy's near drowning. Cynthia, Bessie and Daisy hung on her every word. Captain McCloy was tall, handsome and strong, with an athletic physique. He didn't look like the kind of man who could be easily swept out to sea. They had not realised until that day how dangerous the currents at Paris Plage could be. Cynthia, who was an excellent swimmer, was quite alarmed by

---

* Lieutenant Hine and Captain Coe later received certificates for their bravery. These were presented to them on 9 December 1916 by Lord Ranfurly.

Lily's tale, since she often bathed in the exact same spot. Vowing to only go for a paddle in future, she patted her pillows to settle down for an early night. The others chatted quietly for a while until lights out and then went to sleep on top of their beds. It was far too hot and sticky to sleep between sheets.

Somewhat energised by her time off, Lily went to work as usual the following morning. In recent weeks, nurses' tasks had become more interchangeable. Quibbles about nurse status and who was allowed to do what job had subsided somewhat in the face of overwhelmingly heavy workloads. Lily thought they would probably surface again once casualty levels became more manageable. But for now at least, Lily was enjoying more variety in her working day. She did complicated wound dressings as a matter of course and was often assigned a seriously ill patient to look after for the duration of her duty time. Dora Little showed her how to barrier nurse patients who were in quarantine, and Elsie Goodman guided her in the art of taking accurate observations. Not all sisters were willing to teach extra nursing skills to VADs, but it made perfect sense to do so.

On 23 August six cases of tetanus were diagnosed. Two of these patients died within a matter of hours. All these cases had open wounds and came down the line from the same casualty clearing station. Consequently military authorities were warned to take urgent precautions against a possible epidemic.

In addition to tetanus cases, Sister Swann, who had recently arrived in Étaples from India, turned out to be suffering from malaria. Several staff members were also infected with mumps. All of these infectious patients needed to be barrier nursed to prevent the spread of disease. Furthermore, most victims of the Somme had sustained multiple wounds, so the number of dressings had trebled. Trained sisters were already struggling to keep on top of their assigned work; this struggle was only alleviated by experienced VADs instructed in certain nursing techniques.

Such rudimentary instruction, however, was not enough in the long term. Medical practice was changing on a weekly basis, and nurses needed to keep abreast of new trends. St John's was at the forefront of medical research, having established a medical research society from the outset. Nevertheless, not everyone was in agreement as to which treatments were best. Captain Hope (later Major) of St John's favoured glycerine wound dressings for instance, whereas other surgeons favoured small gauze bags packed with sphagnum moss or pine sawdust. The cost of dressings also varied considerably, and it was difficult to predict quantities needed. An article written by Sir A. Ogston and L. J. Maxse Esquire highlighting this problem was published in *St John's Gazette* in August 1916:

Students of military surgery must contemplate with bated breath the prospects of the next six months of the war.

Including all combatants, there are some thirty millions of men who will, in that period, be more or less exposed to the hazard of accidents, diseases and wounds. The crisis of the contest has now been reached, the stake has to be won or lost, and nothing which our minds can at present conceive will delay or avert the price which has to be paid for the decision. It is the cost incurred by some nations of the world by reason of their ambitions on the one hand and their unpreparedness on the other.

Although we possess no exact statistics bearing on the point, it may safely be concluded that the average minimum number of dressings per man which will be required is at the very least thirty. This means that at least 100,000 dressings will be needed over the next six months.

Trimble and his quartermaster spent considerable time costing supplies, but hospital surgeons would often take it upon themselves to buy dressings locally. Glycerine was in short supply, yet Captain Hope still managed to buy a six-month supply locally for the sum of £42. St John's surgical team were like a close-knit family, headed by Chief Surgeon Major Maynard Smith, a tall, strapping fellow with a big booming voice. Maynard was also a gentle, kindly man who always put the needs of his patients first. However, on 20 August, Trimble received a letter from Sir Arthur Sloggett informing him of Maynard Smith's promotion to the position of Consultant Surgeon to the British Forces in France. Trimble was somewhat dismayed, and on receiving this news he wrote:

> I regret exceedingly that he is severing his connection with the hospital for two reasons. Firstly, he is an especially brilliant surgeon, and secondly he is an excellent companion. However, I am glad his services have been recognised, because he richly deserves his promotion.

Captain Hope succeeded Maynard Smith as chief surgeon, and the latter was given an exceptionally well-attended leaving party. Silently grieving the loss of his excellent companion, Trimble buried himself in his work. Very soon, his mind was taken over by mundane hospital matters. He wrote on 30 August:

> The weather here during the last two days has been exceedingly tempestuous with thunderstorms and torrential rain, which has rather interfered with our sewage outfall works, however, we are grappling with the problem and I do not anticipate any great trouble in this direction.

Sewage problems were resolved in a matter of days. This was just as well, because a new convoy of seventy-two patients arrived from No. 28 ambulance train on 31 August. Staff watched intensely as the train disgorged its bundles of severely injured men, over 80 per cent of them requiring urgent operations. Lily noted in a letter to Agnes:

Everyone is always a bit nervy and agitated when a convoy first arrives, but they soon settle, and teams of medical and nursing staff very quickly get on with the job. We find numerous shell shocked men amongst the wounded. Managed to get to bed by 4am.

Once patients were bedded down nurses could conduct their wards according to normal routines. Much depended on when convoys arrived. For example, on several occasions men did not get their baths if a convoy arrived mid-morning. However, most convoys arrived during the night straight from the front line. Nurses simply had to grab some sleep as and when they were able. When told to expect a convoy or informed that 'a big push' was imminent, over 50 per cent of nurses chose to sleep in their uniforms. This saved them a good deal of time, as they were ready to deal with patients as soon as they were awoken.

Yet a lack of sleep and grim workloads were not allowed to dominate every aspect of a nurse's life. Concerts, plays, sports days and other recreational activities were part and parcel of life. Morale was important, as were social occasions such as birthdays, anniversaries, religious festivals and interpersonal relationships. In the sisters' mess in late August, for example, a discussion was in full swing as to what wedding gift should be bought for Captain Brunwin and his bride-to-be, Bessie Trimble. Silver candlesticks, a silver photo frame, a silver cruet set, a fruit bowl and some bed linen were all put forward as suitable presents for the happy couple.

Meanwhile, Bessie, bubbling with excitement, was regaling her friends with details of her wedding plans. Everything was now arranged; her wedding gown was being made by a dressmaker friend of her future mother-in-law, and her flowers were to be supplied by a Kensington florist. Captain Brunwin had bought her wedding ring and organised their reception. Bessie promised to save a piece of wedding cake for all of her nursing friends, because she knew that most of them would not be able to attend the wedding. Much would depend on convoys, numbers of patients and types of injuries. Bessie was determined, however, to make the most of her wedding day, in spite of limitations imposed by war.

Colonel Trimble was also looking forward to his daughter's wedding. He liked and approved of Alan Brunwin, a determined, principled young officer with a strong sense of responsibility. His attention to the welfare of his men also endeared him to the commanding officer, and Trimble considered him to be a most suitable match for his daughter. He was not overly fond of the paraphernalia that seemed to surround wedding arrangements, since he viewed this to be a woman's domain, but nevertheless listened with interest when his daughter informed him of her preparations, and her happiness gave him great comfort.

11

Fighting on the Somme reached a new intensity in early September. Official communiqués published in the *British Courier* newspaper and elsewhere on 7 September 1916 described the situation as follows:

> Desperate fighting on the Somme
>
> To the north of the Somme there was a violent struggle, without infantry action. To the south of the Somme in the afternoon our troops resumed their offensive action with success. We have captured several German trenches to the south east of Belloy-en-Santerre.
>
> An official communique received today confirms that north of the Somme the enemy did not attempt any counter attack in the night. The artillery struggle continues actively on different sections of the front. South of the Somme the Germans several times attacked our positions south of Deniecourt and in the neighbourhood of Berny-en-Santerre. All those attacks were smashed under our curtains of fire, and cost the enemy losses.

However, another article in the same paper was relatively upbeat about the situation:

> Extension of activity to sectors north of the Somme may be prelude to fresh attack.
>
> Sir Douglas Haig has distributed his artillery bombardments and gas discharges over a very wide area, as anyone may see who takes the trouble to refer back to

the British communiques circulated during the last two or
three weeks.

The enemy are being continually harassed all the way from
the sea to the Somme. Gommecourt is in German hands, the
British line sweeping round immediately to the west of it.

Newspaper reports could only publish heavily censored
extracts of official communiqués. They were not allowed to
report on staggering casualty figures or on the huge loss of life.
Neither could they go into detail with regard to new weapons
technology, since these reports could fall into enemy hands and
undermine military operations.

Chemical warfare as a weapon, for example, had long been the
subject of medical research. Before 1916, gas victims, who gasped
for breath in crowded wards of base hospitals, were simply made
as comfortable as possible until they died. A few men did survive,
but they were left with severely impeded lung function. A British
physician named J.S. Haldane, however, had been working with
C.G. Douglas, L. Hill and J. Barcroft to develop an effective gas
mask, or respirator. Haldane, who had first identified the fact that
Germans were using chlorine and phosgene in their arsenal of
gas canisters, conducted several experiments. Haldane would sit
in a room whilst various gases were poured in through a door.
He would note how these gases affected his brain function and
his respiration. Chlorine and phosgene worked by causing mass
inflammation and irritation of the lungs, which in turn caused
oxygen deprivation. Haldane concluded that lungs affected in
this way needed to be flooded with oxygen as soon as possible
after a gas attack. Subsequently, he constructed special apparatus
designed to administer oxygen to soldiers affected in this way.
Clinical trials were performed on gas victims with encouraging
results, and eventually over 4,000 oxygen cylinders were sent to
base hospitals in France. Thus oxygen therapy became a new and
accepted method of treatment for gas victims. As a consequence,
more men survived chemical warfare.

Practical applications of research findings were usually introduced to base hospitals without deliberation. Moreover, hospital staff were expected to go to lectures promptly to learn new medical or nursing techniques. At busy times Matron selected a few senior nurses to attend such lectures, relying on them to pass on their newly acquired knowledge to their subordinates. Furthermore, when wards were heavy the hectic orderlies often volunteered to take on additional tasks; this was recommended by one hospital orderly named Wilson Crewdson, who wrote:

> Now a few suggestions as to how men attached to hospitals as orderlies, can, in addition to their regular work, assist the sisters and V.A.D. nurses. To carry the food to the various wards and, as far as possible, assist in its distribution is a small matter that will suggest itself to everyone; but it may not at first be quite so obvious that in each ward there is throughout the day a constant accumulation of pails containing discarded dressings, all more or less septic, which require emptying and disinfecting. An inquiry at regular times in the ward will save many a struggle to a hard worked nurse, who will bravely struggle with these heavy weights if left to herself.

Somme battles ensured that wards continued to be full, heavy and hectic. Men who were admitted straight from the battlefield arrived with no field card giving details of age, regiment or seriousness of wounds. They were instantly assessed upon arrival, and over 90 per cent of them needed urgent, life-saving operations. Thus surgical wards in particular had a very high turnover, frequently evacuating up to 230 men in an evening to make way for fresh casualties, who could number 400 or more and invariably arrived in the night. Yet nurses still took the time to befriend each patient. During a lull between convoys of incoming wounded, patients sometimes had the opportunity to offload their troubles to nursing staff. Elsie noted during her spell of night duty:

> A very nice boy Lt. MacClean came in. He was at Toronto University but lives further west. Spent most of his time in the States. A down, morose kind of moody boy at intervals, but clever and nice to talk to. Thinks out things all the time and is a student of philosophy. He slept badly so I used to have long talks with him and missed him when he went.
>
> I came on duty in L ward. I am very sorry for lots of things, there is no doubt it is a test occasionally. Very heavy ward, I've men with gas gangrene.
>
> Lt. Wilson died in the night. His wife arrives tomorrow. Poor thing, so awful for her, and going back alone too. Later Captain Johnson died, also a Canadian regiment.

Elsie, whose arrival had caused quite a stir amongst the male hospital staff, was totally devoted to her darling boys. She had an abundance of sympathy and nursed all of her patients with tender kindness. A string of admirers attempted to court her affections when she first arrived, but Elsie only consented to take tea with the padre. It was important to set the tone of her assignations from the outset. A nurse, trained or otherwise, needed to guard her reputation. Moreover, Elsie was generally dismissive of courtship rituals and flirtatious behaviour. However, in the early days of September a secret admirer began leaving gifts at Elsie's door. Each evening when she awoke from her daytime slumber, she was greeted with small posies of wild flowers, boxes of chocolates, carefully wrapped pieces of cake or bottles of scent. The latter gift in particular was much appreciated and shared with other nursing sisters. Nursing staff were not allowed to wear make-up, but they were allowed to wear scent. In part because it was important to smell nice when nursing the men, but also because it helped to mask the stench of gangrenous wounds. As Elsie's gifts continued to arrive with dependable regularity, her curiosity was aroused. She tried to wake up earlier in the day, hoping to catch her admirer in the act, but to no avail. Eventually she enlisted the help of several other sisters and VADs, all of whom promised to keep a look out for the gift bearer. Romantic intrigue was a welcome diversion from ordinary routine.

Sister Templeton, meanwhile, was in the process of galvanising support to undermine Matron's nurse rotation policy. She bustled down corridors and inspected wards, while all the time planting seeds of discontent. Several sisters who were reluctant to leave their comfort zone in order to move around wards initially gave their backing to Templeton's efforts, although the majority of sisters remained loyal to Matron. Furthermore, even those sisters who expressed sympathy with Templeton were not prepared to do so openly. It was one thing to voice an opinion, but it was quite another to flagrantly oppose Matron.

Templeton nonetheless continued to pursue her goal with tenacity. Like a dog with a bone, she was determined to get her own way. Having been let down by the nursing staff, she started to work on the medical staff. Whenever the chance arose she would ask medical officers if she could have a quiet word in their ear. Other times she would invite them to tea, explaining that she had something most urgent to discuss with them. She told senior medical officers that she was terribly concerned about patient care. The practice of moving sisters around the wards, she informed them, was detrimental to patients because it undermined continuity of care. Furthermore, according to Templeton, patients were suffering dreadfully at the hands of nurses who were inexperienced in certain specialities. Naturally alarmed by such information, medical officers gradually began to question existing nursing policy. Templeton was also politically astute and vented her views especially to the newly promoted chief surgeon, Captain Hope. It was only a matter of time before things would come to a head.

Across the dry-looking lawns, Colonel Trimble was bent over his paper work. He was aware of the strained relationship which existed between Matron and her assistant but unaware of distinct policy clashes. He was about to go on leave to attend his youngest daughter's wedding, and clearing his desk was uppermost in his mind. He simply wanted to tidy up all loose ends before handing over temporary command to Major Houston from the pathology laboratory. He had two new memos to write. The first memo was a warning with regard to hawkers selling their wares to convalescent patients:

> Troops are warned against purchasing fruit and ice creams from hawkers. The articles sold by these people cannot be supervised properly. They are frequently kept for some time under very dirty conditions, and much of the fruit is washed in water, which is probably infected, before being exposed for sale. Ice creams are especially dangerous as the ingredients used are very liable to infection by germs of disease. Many of the cases of disease which occurred in autumn of last year originated in the eating of bad fruit.

The second memo was a standing orders amendment number 1401, which referred to the possession of alcohol:

> Paragraph 8, as amended by routine order 143 of 1916 is cancelled and the following substituted: –
>
> Alcohol. (a) The sale of alcohol is prohibited by law, and any Warrant Officer (W.O.) or Non Commissioned Officer (N.C.O.) or man buying any sort of spirituous liquer renders himself liable to prosecution and punishment. No W.O., N.C.O., or man is to be in possession of any sort of spirituous liquers.
>
> (b) Spirits shall only be sold for consumption by officers, and all orders for such shall be in the form of bulk orders on the nearest Expeditionary Force Canteen (E.F.C.)

Branch. No spirits will be allowed to be sold by the E.F.C. to Sergeant's messes.

(c) As regards to Officer's messes. The voucher will be signed by a staff officer of headquarters in Etaples.

(d) Ordinary Red and White wine, beer and cider, are not included in the term 'alcohol'.

According to this memo, only spirits came under the umbrella term of alcohol, a distinction that gave amusement to many of the men who subsequently read it.

His desk cleared, Trimble wandered thoughtfully along the gravelled walkways to the officers' mess. He knew that he could only be away for a few days, and he prayed that all would be well during his absence. His suitcase was already packed. He and his daughter would travel to Boulogne, stay there for one night and catch the boat across the Channel in the morning. Captain Alan Brunwin had travelled the previous day. He was eager to double-check all wedding arrangements and try on his new suit for size.

Bessie could hardly contain her excitement. She had carefully wrapped her delicate wedding trousseau, placing it uppermost in her suitcase to minimise creasing. Lily, Cynthia, Daisy and Emma had managed between them to buy an exquisite silver photograph frame. Nursing sisters Dora Little, Jane Bemrose, Margaret Ballance and Bertha Smith presented her with some elegant silver candlesticks. Matron had organised a collection amongst all staff, and with funds raised she had bought the practical present of some high-quality bed linen and a round, white tablecloth made of Nottingham lace.

During the past ten weeks Bessie had only been able to snatch a few hours with her fiancé. They had managed three picnics in the woods, five strolls along Cecil Plage beach and two assignations for afternoon tea in Étaples. Many of their planned activities were cancelled at the last minute because of the unpredictability of convoy arrivals. Bessie was therefore

thrilled to be going home on leave. Finally, she would be able
to spend some uninterrupted quality time with her intended.
Her only concern was the boat trip across the Channel. She was
not a natural sailor and usually felt queasy before they even left
the harbour. Her father, however, relished the journey. He loved
the bracing sea air, the rhythmic sway of the boat and, most of
all, his first sighting of the English coast.

Knowing his daughter's tendency towards seasickness,
Trimble considerately read to her throughout the crossing.
He firmly believed that her sickness would subside if her
attention was diverted. He picked several articles which he
found amusing, like the following written by a hospital orderly
in France:

> We all admire the trim grace which regulates the appearance
> of the working girl in France. Her clothes seem to fit like the
> sails of a well-found yacht. Our British girls now have the
> chance of wearing the uniform of the St John and the British
> Red Cross Society, or the brown general service uniform of
> the kitchen or parlour staff. There is nothing as charming as
> a nice print dress, and whether she be from Great Britain
> or the Greater Britain beyond the seas, the V.A.D. knows
> what a becoming dress is, and sees that it fits and is clean and
> smart as clever fingers can make it. Such is the effect of this
> uniform that she is at once able to compete with her French
> sister in smartness of appearance. The head-dress is always
> becoming, especially when worn by the sister, when in a
> curious way it recalls the pictures of the dignified dames of
> Plantagenet times.

Momentarily Bessie smiled, wondering how Matron would
react if someone suggested that uniforms should fit her nurses
like a well-found yacht. Trimble also chuckled. The very idea
that British nurses should somehow have to compete with
French sisters over their appearance was nonsense. As if they

didn't have anything more important to do. It was laughable to the extreme. He wondered if this particular orderly was living in a fantasy land.

The crossing was calm and uneventful. Bessie and her father were greeted by family members, friends and, of course, Captain Brunwin. Panicked by the strength of the welcome home party, Bessie suddenly had an attack of nerves. Perhaps she would trip as she walked down the aisle. Maybe her face would break out in spots on the big day. There could be a Zeppelin raid when the service was in full swing. She had eaten heartily during the past few weeks, so perhaps her dress would be too tight. Perhaps it would pour with rain. Beset with hundreds of 'ifs' and 'maybes', Bessie was relieved when she finally reached home. In her own bedroom, surrounded by her own possessions, she felt safe and secure. She prayed long and hard that evening, asking God to take away her anxieties. In the morning she felt refreshed and thankful. Talking with her capable mother and older sister, Harriet, over breakfast, Bessie regained her usual equilibrium. There was nothing for her to worry about, everything was organised with military precision. There were two days to go, and her mother had arranged two shopping trips, a dress fitting for Bessie and her bridesmaids, and a lovely luncheon beside the river. After the long, sometimes sombre weeks of tending to the injured, Bessie was at last able to relax.

12

Bessie awoke on her wedding day, 16 September 1916, to glorious sunshine. Sounds of clinking crockery and smells of toasted bread drifted up to her room. She stepped out of bed to look tentatively in her dressing table mirror and, with a sigh of relief, she noted her complexion was clear. Then her bedroom door was flung open by Harriet, who bounced on her bed and told her to hurry downstairs. Bouquets of flowers were delivered early, and the whole living room resembled a florist shop. Soon the house was full of animated people. With feelings of elation, Bessie moved from room to room, to be enthusiastically greeted by well-wishers, some of whom were neighbours, who had just 'popped in' to see the bride. Harriet gave them all a brief opportunity to speak to Bessie before ushering them gently out of the house.

A flurry of activity ensued. Breakfast was eaten, crockery washed and cleared away. The bridesmaids, two pretty little girls who were allowed to run around the gardens for a while before putting on their dresses and mob caps, arrived mid-morning. Because she had already been a bridesmaid on three occasions, Harriet had declined to be a bridesmaid to her sister. 'Always the bridesmaid, never the bride' was a popular saying, and she was very superstitious. It was what her mother called 'an old wives' tale', but Harriet was taking no chances.

Colonel Trimble retreated to the drawing room whilst everyone else was getting ready. There he waited patiently until the bathroom was free and the babble of voices subsided. Once his womenfolk were dressed in their finery, he made an appearance. They looked wonderful: his wife was in navy blue, his eldest daughter in blue silk and his youngest in the most beautiful white chiffon wedding gown. Trimble felt a lump in his throat as he surveyed the scene. His wife smiled and briefly embraced him, before chiding him for not being ready. Trimble was, as usual, unflappable. He had prepared his best uniform, which was pressed and laid out on their marital bed. He merely needed to trim his moustache and comb his greying hair.

As wedding cars came and went, ferrying family members to St Peter's church in Kensington, Trimble stood alone with Bessie for a few treasured moments. As they left for the church the whole street gathered to sneak a peek at the bride and to cheer them on their way. Ten minutes later, as her father walked her down the aisle, Bessie looked towards her bridegroom and felt as though she would burst with happiness. The war could not spoil this day. This was going to be a day of joy and celebration. It was also a day that prompted considerable press attention. Trimble's family were pillars of the local community and very important within the Order of St John of Jerusalem.

Alan and Bessie's wedding ceremony was reported in the press as follows:

The marriage was solemnised on Saturday September 16th at St Peters Cranley Gardens, Kensington, of Captain Alan D. Brunwin, R.A.M.C., son of the late Mr George Alfred Brunwin, of Rayne, and Miss Bessie Brereton Trimble, younger daughter of Lieut-Col. Charles J. Trimble, M.G., R.A.M.C. of Bamber Bridge, Preston, Lancs. The ceremony was conducted by the Rev. Canon Deed. D.D. (uncle of the bridegroom), assisted by the Rev. Claude Trimble. B.A., (cousin of the bride).

The bride, who was given away by her father, was attired in a gown of white chiffon taffetas, covered with very pale pink and white tulle, the bodice being of tulle caught in at the waist by a broad belt of taffetas. She wore a tulle veil, surmounted by a wreath of orange blossom, and she carried a sheaf of lilies. She was attended by two little girls as bridesmaids. Miss Peggy Orr (cousin of the bride) and Miss Molly Biggart (niece of the bridegroom). They wore pretty frocks of pale pink taffeta and georgette trimmed with pretty pink rosebuds and forget-me-nots, and sashes; with cream net mob caps with pink and blue ribbon streamers, and carried bunches of pink roses tied with blue ribbon. Each wore a gold regimental badge brooch, the gift of the bridegroom.

The bride's mother wore a navy blue taffeta coat and skirt trimmed with lemon coloured silk and a black velvet hat with lemon colour wings. She carried a bouquet of yellow roses. The bride's sister was attired in a soft navy blue ribbed silk and chiffon gown, with a cherry coloured hat, and wore a spray of carnations. The bridegroom's mother wore a black satin gown, relieved with old lace, and a black and white hat with white ostrich flume, and carried a bouquet of red roses.

The service was choral, and commenced with the hymn 'Thine for ever, God of love,' followed by the hymn 'Oh perfect love.' The concluding hymn was 'O Father, all creating.' Mr G.E. Brunwin (brother of the bridegroom), acted as best man.

After the ceremony a reception was held at Bailey's Hotel Gloucester Road, and later in the day the bride and groom left for their honeymoon, the bride going away in a grey costume trimmed with pink ribbon.

Alan and Bessie spent a glorious week in Brighton before Alan was required to return to the Brigade Hospital in Étaples. In the meantime, Bessie stayed in Chelmsford to establish their new home. Colonel Trimble travelled back to Étaples with his eldest daughter, Harriet, who was also a VAD nurse with the Order of St John. He was back behind his hospital desk a mere three days after the wedding and wrote with some satisfaction in his weekly report to St John's Gate:

I am glad to be in a position to report that during the pressure everything has worked out quite smoothly. In fact I have the confidence to believe that we could deal with a more intense strain without any inconvenience.

Trimble was preparing for a visit from Lady Perrott. He personally inspected the cleanliness of all wards and departments, which were gleamingly spick and span. Under the spotless exterior, however, there were murmurs of discontent. On 21 September, Trimble wrote wearily in his company orders book, 'I had an interview with matron concerning the disagreement between the assistant matron and herself. This state of affairs has been going on for some time.'

Incensed that Matron had taken the opportunity to discuss their rift with the commanding officer, Sister Templeton pushed Captain Hope into action; after all, she informed him, the situation was now dire. On 23 September, Trimble noted:

I had the matron and Captain Hope in my office. Captain explained certain points regarding the frequent changing of sisters in certain wards.

There is undoubtedly much of what appears to be unnecessary moving of the nursing staff. I pointed out to matron that this was against the interests of the patients and the efficiency of the hospital.

Thus, in one fell swoop, Trimble put an end to Matron's nurse rotation policy. Matron, though greatly disappointed, acquiesced gracefully to his decision. There were times when she felt lonely at the top, as she explained in a letter to her sister Mollie: 'You can't think how dull it is having no-one to discuss anything with, most melancholy.'

Sister Templeton, meanwhile, smugly informed nursing sisters that they would be able to remain on their own wards for the duration of their contracts. Spurred on by her success,

Templeton began to look for other ways of undermining her superior; it seemed she fully intended to continue her vendetta until Matron was pushed out of office. Then, of course, she would be promoted to matron. She simply had to make Matron appear incompetent. Her plans to do this, however, were put on hold as a rush of incoming wounded took priority.

This batch of wounded were different than previous groups. They were nearly all stretcher cases as usual, most of them seriously injured; yet these men were smiling, happy and full of stories of armoured vehicles 'putting the wind up the Hun'. When scraps of information were finally pieced together, it was clear that a new weapon had entered the Somme arena. On 15 September 1916 the tank made its dramatic debut as part of the Somme offensive during the battle of Flers-Courcelette. Two days later *The Manchester Guardian* described its impact:

> The British army has struck the enemy another heavy blow north of the Somme. Attacking shortly after dawn on a front more than six miles north east of Combles. Armoured cars working with the infantry were the great surprise of this attack.
>
> Sinister, formidable and industrious these novel machines pushed boldly into no-mans-land, astonishing our soldiers no less than they frightened the enemy. Walking wounded grinned through their bandages and grinned as they talked of these extraordinary beasts while waiting their turn at advanced dressing stations. Even the stretcher cases chuckled as they lay in the ambulances. I heard a fragment of conversation as a grievously wounded man was lifted out of a casualty clearing station: And he says, 'Lord, there was one of those iron boxes strolling down the high street of Flers like it was Sunday afternoon. The man who invented these new and efficient machines of destruction deserves much of the army, if for no more reason than that he has made us laugh as it fought. Not the laughter of ridicule, but of admiration.'

The tank was initially the brainchild of Lieutenant Colonel Ernest Swinton and was developed in the mechanical warfare department under the guidance of Lieutenant Colonel Albert Stern. The tank was so called in order to maintain secrecy: people discussing tanks appeared to be referring to water containers. These first tanks travelled very slowly and did not achieve very much on their first outing. Forty-nine tanks entered the Somme conflict and less than half reached no-man's-land. Yet in terms of boosting morale, they were a huge hit. Germans panicked at the sight of thundering machine-gun wielding iron vehicles, and they did make some gains. Henceforth the tank became an integral part of the armed forces' weaponry.

Certainly those who were wounded at Flers-Courcelette were overjoyed to have fought alongside these new armoured vehicles. Ten days later, as Lady Ethel Perrott toured the wards of St John's, some of the men were still talking excitedly about these revolutionary machines. During her two day visit, Lady Perrott made a point of talking to every patient, even those who were helpless or morose. She was guided around the hospital by Commanding Officer Trimble and Matron. Since she worked steadfastly fund-raising behind the scenes, Lady Perrott wanted to check how this money was being spent. Beds were sponsored, for example, so she needed to make sure that bed heads were labelled correctly with the appropriate names of sponsors. She also wanted to discuss further fund-raising issues. Lady Perrott had a number of planning meetings with both Trimble and Matron. Together they identified patients' needs and decided that the depot system for the distribution of equipment needed to be expanded. Lady Perrott also offered Matron a much-needed listening ear. Relieved to have someone to talk to, Matron discussed her staffing concerns and discreetly alluded to her ongoing problem with Sister Templeton. Lady Perrott assured Matron that her position was safe. No amount of plotting would fool her.

On her return to England, Lady Perrott wrote a cheerful note to Trimble:

> Just a line!
> I myself have got £625 to send to depot 11.
> I've got nearly all the money needed for Xmas presents and orderlies dinners. Soon I shall get that finished, next week.
> I am sending Miss Hay as the new V.A.D. matron asks for. I believe she is excellent and is keen.
> We shall send presents for staff, money for orderlies dinners, and presents for patients.

September drew to a close as Trimble placed the note carefully in his desk drawer. For now the hospital was quiet, the staff were relatively content and the patients in good spirits. Trimble wondered how long this calm would last.

13

Spurred on by the arrival of tanks, British troops pressed forward in the hope of gaining higher ground, but the weather in October was appalling. Torrential rain flooded the rat-infested trenches, and roads were awash with rivers of chalky mud. Battlefields were transformed from soft, rolling meadows into thick, sticky lakes of sludge. Powerful winds combined with heavy rain impeded British progress, and German counter-attacks ensured that casualty figures remained high. Yet again, injured men were admitted to St John's straight from the front line. Some were brought in by members of the 130th St John Field Ambulance, a front-line unit that saved hundreds of lives. Furthermore, as Trimble noted on 4 October:

> It is perfectly clear the authorities recognise the capability of this hospital to deal with the most severe type of cases, and as the convoys under review demonstrate, most of cases are stretcher. Total number of very seriously wounded was large, many surgical operations necessary.

Seven days later he recorded that 'As is usual types of cases very bad, many being in the worst condition. There were nine fatal cases. Interesting to note that we evacuated three hundred and twenty eight out of three hundred and seventy seven.'

Over the following week another eighteen men died. Not surprisingly, given the serious condition of their patients, death rates at St John's far surpassed those of other base hospitals. Seasoned nursing sisters and VADs coped with the dead and dying compassionately and competently. In addition,

they efficiently nursed their patients with cheery smiles and
words of reassurance. But newly recruited nurses, who were
unaccustomed to working on battle-scarred wards, often found
the pace and nature of the work too much to bear.

Those who could not withstand the pressure were gently
eased out of service. Commanding officer reports indicate that
nurses were allowed at least one breakdown in their mental
health before their contract was terminated:

> Sister Gervine and V.A.D. nurse Reny Taylor were taken into
> the sick sisters' home in Le Touquet. I am greatly afraid that
> the last named lady will have to be invalided to England as
> this is the second breakdown since she came to us a short
> time ago.

Lily, much to her astonishment, had discovered that she was
perfectly able to work under extreme and strenuous conditions.
She had considerably grown in confidence and regularly
undertook tasks that were on a par with probationer nurses in
training. Indeed, when injured men requiring urgent attention
flooded endlessly in, Lily, along with other VADs, did much
the same work as trained nursing sisters. However, in terms of
overall nurse status issues, this situation was problematic. Lily,
Cynthia, Daisy and Emma were all considering a post-war
career in nursing, although they were somewhat deterred by the
prospect of having to start from scratch and train in a civilian
hospital for three years. They believed that their experience in a
front-line hospital should count towards general nurse training.
They were not alone in this belief. A leading article in *The Times*
advocated a more flexible approach towards nurse training:

> These new recruits (V.A.D.s) have not received the full
> three years training, which is considered essential by the
> great hospitals, and therefore, in some areas, friction has
> arisen between them and the fully qualified nurses. This was

inevitable, but it has produced a situation of some delicacy, and to some extent has curtailed the supply. A more important matter is the future of these voluntary nurses. Surgeons and doctors who have had V.A.D. members working under them in military hospitals, make no secret of their desire to employ them after the war. They are very good material, yet it is clear that most of them will have to start on a three years training after having done a year or more in a military hospital. It is suggested that the civil hospitals should allow probationers, who have served in military hospitals, to count part of their time in these hospitals towards a general training. This would be a great inducement to women to begin training as war nurses.

Arthur Dale, editor of *St John Ambulance Gazette*, also endorsed this view:

The professional nurse will, no doubt, look askance at such a proposal as this, but the war has wrought great changes in this as in other professions. We realise that it is not desirable to lower the standard of training or to hinder the progressive developments in the system of training for nurses which has taken place of recent years, and we do not think this proposal will in any way do so, providing that the members of the V.A.D.s who have worked continuously for two years in an auxiliary military hospital, with no less than six hours duty per day count these two years towards their training as trained nurses, undergoing a period of special training to make up for the three years of the probationary period.

Predictably, trained nurses were highly suspicious of any attempt to dilute professional nursing with scarcely trained VADs, regardless of their individual merit. Moreover, such attempts as there were merely fuelled the drive towards nurse registration. VADs, meanwhile, were not as politically aware, and most of them were not overly concerned with their career prospects. A marriage bar* was in existence, which required all women to give up their employment as soon as they were married. Most young women were eager to marry, establish a home and have children. If there was a straightforward choice between marriage and career, the former usually took precedence. Unmarried women were often pitied for being 'on the shelf' and expected to stay at home to care for elderly relatives. Those who were committed to a religious calling or a vocation such as nursing, however, commanded respect rather than pity.

Lily and her friends wanted to fall in love, to be whisked off their feet, to experience a whirlwind romance. They chatted about members of the opposite sex, and in particular they discussed the merits of individual officers: those who had nice smiles, those who were shy, those who were amusing and witty, those who were handsome and those who were dark and brooding. But as yet they had not formed any romantic attachments. They had, however, along with some of the sisters, been enlisted by Elsie to track down her secret admirer. To date they had narrowed the list down to medical officer Lieutenant Jackson, Major Houston, Captain Hope and Chef Marco, although Lily only suspected the latter because he had unlimited access to cake and other foodstuffs. Spying on the male staff was proving to be rather more difficult than expected. Elsie remained optimistic that her admirer would eventually be revealed, but she confessed to her spies that she didn't really find any of the shortlisted men in the least bit attractive. She continued to keep tabs on her darling boys, however, writing in her diary:

> I've just heard that Jack McClean has been wounded again and was at No.2 Red Cross hospital in Rouen, but went to Blighty [England] on the tenth. Poor boy it is bad luck.

---

* The marriage bar was finally lifted during the Second World War.

> We have a Lieut. Harris from Vancouver in just now, a nice
> youth. Captain Frenchman of L ward and Major Jones of
> London Regiment, all very nice. One wonders whether one
> will ever come across these people again.

Elsie was totally devoted to her patients and enjoyed good
relationships with both medical and nursing staff. But she was
astute enough not to get drawn into nursing politics. She refused
to become involved in Sister Templeton's feud with Matron, for
example, claiming that her only interest was the welfare of the
men in her care, although Templeton's simmering machinations
soon became a matter of general concern. Sisters Jane Bemrose,
Ida Bull, Molly McGinnis, Dora Little and Catherine Warner
began to argue forcefully against Templeton's views. There
was something rather distasteful, they argued, about involving
medical officers such as Captain Hope in nursing policy. Then
they pointed out to other members of the nursing staff that
during the previous March, 41 per cent of the nursing staff were
off sick. Obviously, therefore, Matron's policy had been correct,
since it made sense to educate sisters as far as possible in all
nursing specialities. The majority of nurses agreed. The tide of
opinion was turning in Matron's favour. Very soon the backlash
against Templeton gathered momentum, and by mid-October
her position was rapidly becoming untenable.

On 25 October Lady Perrott made another brief visit to
St John's, which gave Matron additional support. Inspecting the
names of bed heads, she wrote enthusiastically:

> Sometimes a patient will be delighted to find that his bed
> or one close to him has been given by some town he knows
> well, or where he has relations. I think that the fact of
> these beds being endowed from every part of the Empire
> serves to show our splendid soldiers how many at home,
> both in England and in our overseas Dominions are caring
> for them.

Over one is a shield stating that this bed has been given by the children of Halifax. These children gave up their prizes one Xmas so that the money might go to help their bed, and they entirely collected the amount with which to endow it.

I am sure that many a wounded hero has felt joy in reading the inscription over his bed.

As Lady Superintendent in Chief, Lady Perrott's visits never failed to boost morale. She praised the splendid work of the nurses and went out of her way to speak to everyone. She valued the importance of good steady leadership and the need for hospital members to work as a team. Current dissension in the nursing ranks was disquieting, and certain issues needed to be resolved. Colonel Trimble had access to an unfettered supply of information with regard to nursing concerns – one of the many advantages of having a VAD daughter. He was also aware of the rumblings and mutterings of complaint against Templeton, which were getting louder by the day. For example, sisters were getting weary of receiving conflicting orders from Matron and Templeton on a daily basis. Matron would arrive on the wards and give an order for all windows to be opened to enable soldiers to breathe in fresh air. Ten minutes later Templeton would arrive on the exact same wards and issue an order for all windows to be closed because she thought there was a chill in the air. This degree of pettiness was tiresome to say the least. Sisters had enough work to do without having to comply with contradictory orders from two superiors who were permanently at loggerheads with each other.

Trimble organised another meeting with Matron in an attempt to resolve this situation. Matron stated her case clearly. As far as she was concerned, there were no problems within the nursing ranks until Templeton was promoted to assistant matron. Templeton, she argued, had proved to be a disruptive influence. Trimble was inclined to agree. Following a long discussion, both he and Matron decided that Templeton needed to be replaced as soon as possible. Trimble promised to ask Lord Ranfurly if he could have permission to secure the services of Matron's close friend Sister Mabel Chittock, who had been with the hospital at its inception. In the meantime, Matron was instructed to speak to all members of her nursing staff to clarify the fact that her orders alone were to be implemented, and they were not to be undermined by anyone. Templeton's influence was immediately curtailed and her orders effectively bypassed during the coming weeks. Further opportunities for pettiness were also limited as the hospital entered a particularly busy period.

Throughout October 1916, 1,417 cases, all with horrendous injuries, passed through St John's. Incoming wounded were caked in mud, splattered with blood and hypothermic. They had advanced in thick mud, plodding against sheets of rain and forceful winds. Weighed down by heavy backpacks, they were totally exhausted when they reached a barely visible front line. They continued to struggle wearily but purposefully towards the enemy and were blown to smithereens by a barrage of artillery fire. One officer recalled being blown into the air before landing in a partially flooded shell crater. He strived to rescue one of his men who had quickly slipped into a muddy quagmire, holding his hand as firmly as he could. Try as he might, he could not save him. His body slipped slowly away, his throat gurgling mud as he drowned. Another officer managed to save two of his men but a third drowned in a similar incident. Yet another held his badly injured friend above water for two hours before help arrived. One young soldier, merely a lad, was sent out to deliver a message to an officer less than 100yds away. He staggered in the slimy mud and was blown off course by the battering winds. He was discovered four days later, dead at the bottom of shell hole. Padres were yet again burying over 100 dead soldiers a day. Other men were already buried alive or missing in action. Apparently some ground had been gained, but it was difficult to tell in the abysmal weather conditions. Soldiers who survived the battle were grieving the loss of their chums. Those who arrived at the hospital were filthy, tired, bewildered and desolate. It took several orderlies all their strength to prise their boots off.

Nurses were run ragged, and surgeons operated on the wounded day and night. Frequently surgeons were forced to operate by candlelight as main lights were turned off for hours when Zeppelins were overhead. The number of fatalities continued to rise. Some staff members were on the point of physical collapse. Yet they pushed themselves ever onwards, dealing with casualties who had sustained the worst wounds they had ever seen. The pressure of work was relentless.

Concerned that his staff might be buckling under such a busy and grim period, Trimble did his best to shore up morale. He organised numerous dances, concerts, plays and chess tournaments. For most staff members these social occasions provided happy and relaxing interludes, as Elsie recorded in her diary: 'October 31st – All Hallows Eve and a little party in the mess room. Very enjoyable too, the best I've had. Began dancing again and find that I'm not as bad as I thought.' But a few did not have the energy to socialise, as Cynthia noted in her diary, 'I am quite simply too tired to go out!'

As part of his efforts to improve morale, Trimble also attempted to gather enough musicians to form a brass band. At this stage a lack of instruments rather than talent prevented this endeavour. However, Trimble was determined. He loved brass bands and had his heart set on establishing a hospital band. This was an ongoing ambition, which met with varying degrees of success in the coming months.

14

Weather conditions deteriorated even further in November. Freezing fog, slate grey skies and drizzly rain spread across the battlefields like a heavy sodden blanket. There was no let-up in the driving winds, and it was almost impossible for soldiers to distinguish the front line. Lily received a letter from Agnes in which she described the fate of their cousin Harry:

> They went into the trenches and were there for some while. They suffered terribly from the cold. Harry amongst others suffered terribly with his feet. They became absolutely numb. At last he asked his officer if he might go sick on account of his feet. The officer refused and said that he couldn't have men going sick because they were foot sore. So he went back to the trenches never questioning his orders. Soon after they came out Harry fell out of line, unable to march. He crawled along and presently an ambulance came up, but there was a worse off man than he to fill the last stretcher. He eventually got to hospital and for months suffered uncomplainingly, even though both his feet were gouged. At nineteen he has been left a cripple.

Lily was distraught. She remembered her cousin as mischievous, handsome, kind and considerate. Now he was unable to walk, toes amputated because of frostbite and his feet distorted. She knew that cases such as these were widespread, but this did not lessen the impact of her sister's letter. Trench foot was caused by soldiers standing for hours in freezing cold water, and as winter set in the condition became a common occurrence.

On 13 November it snowed heavily all day. A severe ground frost over the next few nights made fighting all the more treacherous. St John's was also affected by the severe weather as water pipes froze and fuel prices rose. But still the battered, war weary wounded spilled through the doors in their hundreds.

In his weekly report to Lord Ranfurly dated 8 November 1916, Trimble gave some indication of admission numbers from the start of the Somme offensive onwards:

> In July, August, September and October 5,202 cases were admitted, whereas from the date of opening to June 30th 6,545 cases were dealt with. The contrast of the work done in the four months and during ten months is very marked. In giving you these figures will you allow me to say that they are for your own private reflection?

These figures reveal an average patient intake of 1,300 patients per month over a four-month period. November figures were slightly lower, with 883 patients admitted. Of these, 833 were stretcher cases and fifty were walking wounded. Workloads remained heavy, therefore, because of stretcher to walking wounded ratios. Staff continued to be placed under extreme pressure, and there were signs that this stress was beginning to take its toll. On 7 November Captain Hope, who had recently been promoted to the rank of major, succumbed to a particularly severe strain of influenza. He was admitted to hospital along with Lieutenant Henry, Captain Coplestone, eight orderlies and ten sisters. Those who worked in the operating theatre or on surgical wards were the most likely to get ill. Sister Kane, a slim attractive brunette who had worked at St John's from the outset, became very ill with rheumatism. Twenty-three other sisters were off sick with septic fingers and thumbs.

Months of overwork and sleep deprivation also affected staff in other ways. Extreme tiredness sometimes led to carelessness. A distressed Elsie noted with great shame in her diary:

November 8th

Came on duty feeling quite happy until 9pm. Then came the biggest mistake of my nursing career and such a one as might have been an awful tragedy, and as such I want to hold it in part of me as an awful lesson all my life against carelessness.

Such kindness I have received from colleagues in spite of it. I couldn't have conceived of, and will never forget. Fortunately for me it didn't end disastrously, and I feel most gratefully for this all of my days. Sister Stinsie came over this morning but I was beyond talking to her. I never want to forget this; and yet I do trust I may soon get back my nerve.

Elsie had made a drug error. Sisters in charge of wards were totally responsible for measuring drug doses and for their administration. When working under severe pressure or suffering from a lack of sleep, mistakes were easy to make. They could also be lethal. For a long time after this event Elsie suffered periodically from nightmares. However, sisters were naturally sympathetic towards Elsie's plight: they understood that no one was infallible. Many told Elsie of their own blunders. One sister had used the wrong dressing solution for a wound, while another had forgotten to apply a poultice. Lily told Elsie of the time she had started bed bathing one gentleman when she was called away to get another man a drink. En route to the kitchen someone else asked her to help lift a patient up to the bed, and she totally forgot about the first gentleman. Twenty minutes later she suddenly remembered him and hastily returned to his bedside – he was still covered in a soapy lather.

Encouraged by Lily and others, Elsie began to slowly regain her confidence. The mystery of her secret admirer was also revealed. Lily pointed out excitedly that since Major Hope had been confined to the officers' ward with flu the flow of small gifts had stopped. Elsie was not convinced, however, until Major Hope recovered and small boxes of chocolates began arriving at her door once more. Elsie noted, 'We conclude that the chocolates are from Major Hope.'

Although the mystery was solved, Elsie chose not to confront Major Hope. She did not reciprocate his affections and did not want to embarrass him. Lily, whose romantic inclinations thrived on notions of happy endings, was bitterly disappointed.

Whilst nurses struggled with mounting fatigue, troops struggled with worsening weather. Snow and freezing fog had transformed shrouded battlegrounds into precarious territory: jagged, shell holed areas littered with barbed wire and debris. Dangerous weather conditions combined with increasing sickness levels prevented further advances. Therefore, on 18 November, the Somme offensive drew to a close. The Allies had gained a mere 6 miles of land. British casualties numbered 432,000, of these 150,000 had died and over 100,000 were severely incapacitated. During the first two weeks of November large numbers of wounded soldiers were admitted to St John's, but towards the end of the month there was a sharp increase in medical cases. These were primarily trench foot, nephritis, bronchitis, lumbago and venereal disease. Furthermore, the issue of malingering surfaced once more, and medical articles were written to give guidance on catching 'skrimshankers'. One such article described how such men complaining of lumbago (muscle pain) could be exposed:

> First of all, let me say that lumbago, the ancient and time honoured raison d etre for getting a few days off duty, is utterly played out. The hardened M.O. regards that word on a report with the utmost scepticism, and, moreover, to act the part needs far more skill than the average recruit possesses. You must wince with pain at the proper moment; this is a sine qua non. There is also a very effective trap for lumbagoists. The M.O. listens to you with almost a bedside manner; he is sympathetic and kindly, and even suggests hospital. No hint of incredulity betrays itself on his features; you are disarmed.

As you turn to go, however, he clumsily drops something at your feet, a stethoscope or coins perhaps. In courtesy you bend down and pick them up. This is fatal and betrays you; his manner changes from that of a courtly physician to one more reminiscent of chief mate of an Atlantic tramp. Your report is marked 'D' and you go back a sadder and wiser man.

In terms of diagnosing and treating sick soldiers, doctors were often required to adopt the role of detective. Some conditions were easier than others to mimic, but if there was any hint of malingering then soldiers were simply sent back down the line.

Treatment of venereal disease (VD) was also a common problem. If men suffering from the disease had reached a stage when treatment was of no use, they were also sent back down the line. Soldiers were five times more likely to be admitted to hospital with VD than with trench foot, but the former was difficult to treat and even more difficult to control. Rates of VD were highest within Canadian forces, with almost a third of soldiers infected with the disease. By comparison the rate within the British army was approximately 5 per cent. British soldiers were encouraged to be chaste, and educated at length about the perils of catching the disease. Indeed, within the British army, control over sexual urges was viewed as a matter of a soldier's honour. In terms of military law it was not a crime to contract the disease, but it was a crime to conceal it. Soldiers with VD, however, were not paid whilst they were receiving medical treatment: a situation that encouraged its concealment. Moreover, young, sexually inexperienced soldiers were frequently tempted to make use of French brothels. They figured that statistically their chances of dying in battle far outweighed the chances of dying of VD. Therefore, they strived to save enough money to visit brothels in order to lose their virginity. Brothels controlled by the French government were monitored, and prostitutes working within them were medically examined on a twice-weekly basis. Nevertheless, the delay between catching VD and displaying signs of infection varied considerably depending on whether a sufferer had caught syphilis or gonorrhoea. Many cases of VD remained undiagnosed during asymptomatic, dormant phases of the disease. Therefore, unsuspecting officers, along with their men, could easily be infected by women who believed themselves to free of the disease.

Treatments for the condition were not very successful. Ablution chambers were set up in Britain and France, so that soldiers could be treated with salvarsan. This was an arsenic-based disinfectant solution that worked well if used immediately after sexual intercourse but was ineffective a few days after the event. Soldiers were also reluctant to use ablution chambers. Yet action was urgently needed to stem the numbers of those infected. Four hundred thousand cases of VD were admitted to base hospitals, which resulted in an enormous drain on military resources. Furthermore, attempts to introduce prophylactics to prevent the spread of VD were met with fierce opposition from social purity groups and religious organisations. They argued that the use of prophylactics would encourage moral degeneration and promiscuity. A report published by a Royal Commission on the subject merely advised that education and abstinence were the keys to beating VD.*

For nurses and medical staff VD was a particular problem, since the disease could easily be transmitted by contact with infected bodily fluids. Dressing wounds without using gloves, for example, could infect a nurse through a tiny scratch in the skin. An infected nurse could then unwittingly transmit the disease to others. Where patients had obvious signs of VD, such as syphilitic chancres, precautions were taken. But asymptomatic patients posed a real threat.

---

* In March 1918 an amendment (40d) to the Defence of the Realm Act stated that it was a crime for women infected with VD to have sexual relations with a member of His Majesty's Forces. This regulation, however, was virtually impossible to enforce and prompted a series of protests from women's groups.

Colonel Trimble regularly placed 'maisons de tolerance' on an out of bounds list for officers and men. Moreover, it seems that most complied with his orders. But prostitution was not confined to brothels. Any woman could turn to prostitution and was more likely to do so in times of economic hardship. Individual prostitutes operating from their own homes were not medically examined for VD, and therefore soldiers faced a far greater risk of catching the disease from these women than if they frequented state-controlled brothels.

Prostitution continued to flourish wherever troops were encamped. There was also a thriving trade in black market goods. In an attempt to stamp out black market profiteering, French authorities issued price guidelines for essential foodstuffs.

St John Hospital
The following are the maximum prices for certain goods as fixed by the French authorities. Anyone selling in excess of these prices is liable to prosecution, and the Commandant desires that everyone connected with the British Forces should give every assistance to the French authorities in this matter.

Goods Price (including all taxes)
Frs. Cts. Per kilogram
Table margarine 2. – 70
Cooking margarine 2. – 10
Chicory Beans 1. – 70
Chicory powdered 1. – 50
Refined sugar 1. – 40
Crystallized sugar 1. – 30
Dried Haricot beans 0. – 90
Vegetables (Lingots 0. – 30
& dried onions.
Potatoes per quintal (1cwt)
Frs. Cts.
Yellow from the producer 15 00

From markets & local merchants 20 00
White from the producer 12 00
From markets & local merchants 17 00
Large blue from the producer 10 00
From markets & local merchants 15 00

When obtained from Wholesale Merchants for delivery of
1 Quintal (1cwt)
  Frs. Cts.
  Yellow 16. – 25
  White 13. – 25
  Large Blue 11. – 25
  Fresh Eggs 5 – – 85 for 26
  Preserved Eggs 3 – – 90 for 26

Signed: Eydoux, General
Commanding Region du Nord

Trimble gave one copy of these guidelines to the quartermaster, Lieutenant Hine, and another to the new head chef, Leon Bartone. The previous head chef, H. Marco, had been dismissed on 15 November over some alleged irregularities with food supplies. No official charges were made against him, but with Christmas fast approaching Trimble wanted to make sure that the kitchen was running smoothly.

Elsewhere in the hospital, preparations were being made to stage a Christmas production of Gilbert and Sullivan's *Mikardo*. Captain Beckett from the surgical block was stage manager. Musical conductors and accompanists were Captain Brunwin and Captain Coplestone, assisted by kind permission of Colonel Martin and by members of the convalescent camp orchestra. The cast were as follows:

The Mikado of Japan – Major Hope.
Nanki Poo (his son disguised as a wandering minstrel in love with Yum Yum) – Lieut. Hine.
Ko Ko (Lord High Executioner of Titipu) – Lieut. Wilson.
Pooh-Bah (Lord High of everything else) – Captain Beckett.
Pish-Tush (A noble Lord) – L/Cpl Johnson.
Yum Yum (3 sisters of Ko Ko) – Nurse M. Betey, Nurse E. Turnball-Smith and Nurse E. Herder.
Katisha (an elderly lady in love with Nanki Poo) – Nurse H. Trimble.
Noblemen of Japan –
Captain Gorder, Captain Coe, Reverend F.E.L. Gower, Sgt. Bolton, Corporals Lockier, Sanderson, Topping, Privates Blackburn, Gray, Lounds, McConway, Miller, Murray, Nicholls, Preston, Sowerbutts, Vernon and Wilkinson.

Lily, Daisy and Cynthia helped Sisters Dora Little, Jane Bemrose, Molly McGinnis, Elsie Goodman and Catherine Warner to make costumes. Emma, meanwhile, used her artistic talents to design and paint scenery and props. A team of willing orderlies assisted her in this task. For the next few weeks, St John's recreation room was a hive of activity. Peals of laughter emanated from within, mixed with tuneful voices and brash bold sounds of a large brass band. Every spare moment was spent in stitching fabrics, rehearsing roles, building stage sets and practising musical scores. Members involved decided to call their hospital stage company PUO. Orderlies constructed a stage and Lily along with her friends stifled giggles as they watched rehearsals from the wings. For the first time in a long while they were able to relax and enjoy life.

15

Preparations for Christmas were well underway at St John's by the start of December. Each ward was expected to provide something in the way of entertainment in addition to the usual carol singing and performances planned by the PUO group. Those not directly involved with entertainment schedules were engrossed in making decorations and party crackers. Some of the medical officers, however, were more preoccupied with British politics than they were with the subject of Christmas festivities. According to *The Times* and official communiqués, dramatic political changes were taking place in Britain. Liberal Prime Minister Herbert Asquith, who had taken Britain to war in 1914, had by this time lost the confidence of many in his own party. In 1915 a shortage of artillery shells and other ammunition had led to a high-profile scandal; a barrage of criticism was directed towards Asquith, which resulted in the formation of a ministry of munitions. The introduction of conscription in March 1916 had also split the Liberal party, and many members blamed their leader for the appalling Somme casualties. Moreover Asquith, although intellectually brilliant and a reasonable peacetime prime minister, did not appear to be coping with wartime demands. David Lloyd George, who had been Minister of Munitions and then Secretary of State for War, was, by comparison, a dynamic, energetic personality who possessed a radical but clear vision of how Britain needed to pursue its war effort. Consequently, with the backing of Conservative and Labour party members, Lloyd George ousted Asquith and became prime minister of a coalition government on 6 December 1916.

This political shift seemed to galvanise the population, and Lloyd George did much to streamline production of munitions. He also established a naval convoy system to ensure an uninterrupted supply of foodstuffs and military equipment. Medical officers generally seemed supportive of these changes and were infused with new optimism. Members of the nursing staff were less enamoured with politics, but Sister Dora Little and VAD Cynthia Owen were consoled at least by the notion that Lloyd George supported women's suffrage.

British political changes, however, did not entirely overshadow events at St John's. Indeed, on the evening of 9 December a very special investiture was held at the hospital. On this particular evening something very remarkable occurred – ten VAD nurses, including Lily and Cynthia, were afforded the Insignia of Honorary Serving Sister of the Order of St John of Jerusalem, in recognition of the wonderful work they had performed during the grim and fierce Somme battles. The decoration was awarded by Earl Ranfurly in the presence of several dignitaries: Colonel Trimble; Commandant, Brigadier General Graham Thompson, CB, CMG; Sir George Makin, KCMG, CB, consulting surgeon to the Étaples district; Colonel Carr, CB, consulting physician; Colonel Plomer and Major White of the commandant's staff; Mr Ridsdale, acting commissioner war committee; and the officers commanding and officers of the hospitals at Étaples together with the matrons, trained nurses and VAD members of these institutions.

Colonel Trimble praised the work of the V.A.D.s who were about to be honoured and welcomed Lord Ranfurly and his other distinguished guests. He recounted that his own association with the Order began in 1882, and his long service had only served to strengthen his veneration for the humanitarian work it was doing. It was interesting, he thought, to remember that once more we found ourselves in the closest alliance with the French as we had been during the Crusades, and that the Order was still carrying out the work for which it was founded in the year 1087.

Lord Ranfurly then presented the decoration to the VAD members and said:

> By the request of the Council and Chapter, and with the sanction of His Majesty the Sovereign Head of the ancient Order, I am about to hand to you the Insignia of Honorary Serving Sister. I have to enjoin you with the cross as the sign of man's redemption, and so may you ever remember in your lives that its four arms symbolise the Christian virtues – Prudence, Temperance, Justice and Fortitude; that its points represent the eight Beatitudes which spring from the practice of these virtues. I am about to hand you a cross, its whiteness is the emblem of that purity of life required in those who fight for the defence of the Christian faith and live for the poor and suffering. I desire to point out that His Majesty has signed his sanction for these to be given with his own hand. I wish to hand to you each a prayer of the Order which is given at the same time as the cross.
>
> Lord Ranfurly then went on to say that it had given him great pleasure to have had the privilege of presenting this well-earned decoration. He recalled that it was in the year 1047 that a hospital was first founded by the Order. From those early days the Order of St John had been of greatest service to civilisation. The hospital in which they were now gathered was the best proof that the Order was still doing the work for which it had been originally established, i.e. the caring for the sick and wounded. He wished to emphasize the fact that the Order was very proud of its hospital, and all at St John's Gate were determined to do everything possible to help them keep up the name they had already earned as the best or one of the best hospitals in France.

For the VADs concerned, such an extraordinary acknowledgement of their efforts was a great honour. It was also an astonishing achievement. In one remarkable investiture the Order of St John of Jerusalem had elevated women working in the lowliest of nursing ranks to the rank of trained sisters. Effectively, this award ceremony dramatically overturned traditional methods of measuring nurse status. The status of trained nurses was normally dependent on the elite standing of their training hospital. The Order of St John, however, had awarded an elitist nursing honour to VADs on the grounds of meritocracy. In doing so, emphasis was placed on sound Christian principles and humanitarian endeavour.

Lily had not paid much attention to status issues, but she was delighted to receive such a prestigious award. Somehow, it made all the hardships and deprivations of the previous few months worthwhile. Cynthia was also happy to have received such wonderful recognition, and her only regret was that her father had died before he was able to witness the ceremony. Lily assured Cynthia that her father was always with her in spirit, and they talked in whispers well into the night. They were content. The investiture evening had provided a welcome interlude from routine, along with a lovely spread of food.

Nevertheless, hospital life continued apace. The problems of relentless cold weather were worsened by a blockade at Boulogne Harbour which held up coal supplies. Convoys of soldiers continued to arrive straight from the front. Furthermore, over 90 per cent of stretcher cases were suffering from trench foot. Tiredness hindered work routines; Sister Irwin and Emma Mieville were sent to convalescent home Hardelot for a rest on 13 December. Meanwhile, Sister Jane Bemrose was sent to Villa Tino to have treatment for a septic finger. Thankfully, they recovered quickly and were all discharged after three days.

On 21 December men were entertained to a delicious supper courtesy of Lady Perrott's fund-raising activities. A musical concert followed supper, and the men shouted three cheers for Lady Perrott at the end of the evening. True to her word, Lady Perrott had organised funds for food and presents, for patients and staff. For Colonel Trimble this was his first Christmas as commanding officer, and he wanted to make it as uplifting as possible. In his report he describes the event as follows:

On the evening of the 24th between the hours of 6pm and 8.30pm carols were sang around the gangways of the hospital. This music was particularly well rendered by the medical staff, sisters, V.A.D.s and orderlies and gave considerable pleasure and satisfaction to the patients.

At 2.30am on Christmas Day we received a convoy of one hundred and fifteen cases (60 stretcher cases and 55 walking cases) and this enabled us to begin Christmas Day feeling that we had discharged a certain amount of duty towards the sick and wounded soldiers.

At 11.30am Salvation Army band came into hospital and played in the centre green: they discoursed a programme of sacred music.

At 12.0'clock dinner was served and I took the opportunity of going round each ward and wishing patients compliments of the season, accompanied by Matron, Major Houston, Major Hope, Captain Gordon and the Orderly Officer. The Sergeant Major was also in attendance.

Wards were exceedingly well decorated, more particularly so in the medical division, as Surgeon in Chief rather objected to elaborate and heavy decorations in surgical wards, all the same very great taste and interest was displayed by sisters and V.A.D.s in putting up very appropriate decoration: and really too much credit cannot be given to all those concerned for their very strenuous and successful efforts to cheer up the wounded and sick soldiers who were committed to their charge.

Trimble continued in the same vein for the remainder of his report. He praised the dinner and particularly the excellent plum pudding, which had been provided by the government. All food was apparently supplied by the quartermaster's stores, except for some sausage, which was supplied out of the Order's funds. Specific menus were as follows:

Christmas Day Menus:
Menu for Patients
Breakfast – Boiled smoked ham, boiled egg, coffee or tea, porridge or milk diet.
Dinner – Roast mutton with onion sauce, green peas, potatoes, Christmas pudding with sauce, fruit. Ale, stout or lime juice cordial.
Tea – Lobster, sardines, herrings, sausage. Stewed prunes and custard, jellies, mince pies, bread and butter, jam and honey and tea.
Supper – Cocoa fancy biscuits and cheese.
Sausage is the only article on above list to be provided by the Order of St John.

Menu for Orderlies
Breakfast – Fish, tea, bread and butter, jam and cheese
Dinner – Roast pork and apple sauce, potatoes and cabbage. Christmas pudding and white sauce, oranges and nuts. Beer, coffee and lime juice.
Tea – Bread and butter, sausage, hot mince pies, and sweet cake.
Supper – Cocoa, cheese and fancy biscuits.

Menu for Remaining Staff
Breakfast – Ham, egg, toast, butter and jam
Dinner – Tomato soup, turkey, York ham with bread sauce, boiled chestnuts, Brussels sprouts and potatoes. Christmas pudding with sauce, special Christmas cake and cheese and biscuits. Beer, wine and coffee.

Tea – Bread, butter, jam and honey. Lobster, ham and sausage, mince pies, fancy biscuits, jellies and cake.

Supper – Cocoa, ham, cheese, bread and butter.

After eating their dinner the patients had a rest period followed by a musical concert. Matron had organised a bran tub (lucky dip) for each ward, and entertainment included songs, poetry recitals, comic impressions of staff members, dance displays and a rendition of trumpet music. There were also a number of opportunities for Christian worship and Holy Communion throughout the day. Reverend Gower held five services, at 5.30 a.m., 7 a.m., 8.10 a.m., 10 a.m. and 12 noon. In total, ninety-one people took communion, mostly patients.

When patients had received their gifts it was time for staff to receive their presents from the Order: silver trinket boxes for nurses and silver pencil cases for the medical officers. Then it was time to thank staff members. Once the orderlies had finished their dinner, Trimble addressed them in the dining room of their barracks:

> I spoke a few words to the men and tried to thank them for the assistance they had given me in carrying on the work of the hospital, because there is no denying the fact that our enlisted St John men have turned out excellent orderlies. They are splendid fellows and their conduct has been exemplary, they have done a great deal for our soldiers and it has been done in a most cheerful and self-denying manner, and I am very proud to have such a body of men under my command.

Matron gave a similar thank-you speech to members of her nursing staff and organised a gathering in the sisters' mess on Christmas Day evening. Sister Templeton did not attend. Undeterred, however, Matron spoke to each of her nurses individually, asking about their family members and generally catching up on their news. She liked to know as much as possible about all of her nurses and encourage them at every opportunity. This Christmas she was especially proud that ten of her VADs had been singled out as deserving of an honorary award. This reflected well on the hospital and on her leadership. But there was not much time to dwell on this success, because the hospital was almost full. On 28 December, just as PUO performers were about to stage *The Mikado*, a convoy of seventy-eight patients arrived. The opera was postponed until new patients were assessed and bedded down. Once staged, however, *The Mikado* was a huge success. Trimble recorded with much satisfaction:

> This first performance was entirely in the interests of our patients and any of our trained sisters and V.A.D.s who could attend, I was also able to get into the hall a good many of our orderlies. On Saturday the 30th the opera was again staged, and on this occasion I asked the Commandant and his staff, the O.C.s of the infantry base depots, together with a certain number of trained sisters and V.A.D.s from the various hospitals. The Duchess of Westminster was also present and altogether I had an attendance of about two hundred and twenty. It was a highly appreciative audience and my feeling is that everybody was greatly surprised at what we had to show them. After the performance light refreshments were served in the officers' mess.

Entertainment schedules were very important in maintaining morale, especially when work was heavy, although total December casualty figures stood at 890, only slightly up from November. Furthermore, fortunately for the staff, the ratio of stretcher cases to walking wounded had improved, with 288 walking cases and 602 stretcher cases.

Both Matron and Trimble were relieved that the number of helpless cases were fewer, but they remained concerned about staff sickness levels. Writing with regard to Sister Kane, Trimble noted:

> This sister went to villa Tino suffering from rheumatism on 19th of October and was there until 6th of December. On this date she was transferred to the convalescent home for nurses at Hardelot and on 21st December she was sent down to Mentone where she is at the present time, and I trust she will in the course of a week or two be fit to resume duty. I felt justified in doing everything I could for this sister as she had been out with us from the start and has done excellent work.

Staff sickness was not helped by the coal famine. Small stocks of coal were reserved for patients' wards, but medical and nursing staff frequently had to go without heating. Warm jumpers were placed over nightclothes, with some nurses wearing at least five pairs of socks in bed. Lily complained to Agnes, 'It is impossible to get warm and we are all getting chilblains.'

Agnes sent Lily some woollen mittens and an old overcoat that had been lying in the lost property department of her hospital. But fuel shortages combined with severe frosts began to affect everyone at the hospital. Orderlies were dispatched to cut down tree branches and collect piles of logs to stoke the stoves. The winter of 1916–17 was one of the worst on record. For men still fighting on the front line the days were bad enough – bitter cold, freezing trenches with very little in the way of shelter – but the nights were even more desperate as temperatures plummeted below freezing. In this severe weather many men suffered varying degrees of frostbite. Moreover, the number of medical cases rose steeply as already debilitated men succumbed to a myriad of infections. Mumps, measles, German measles, scarlet fever, tuberculosis, septic throats and influenza became commonplace over the next few months.

16

New Year's Day 1917 was celebrated with a dance in the officers' mess. It was a joyful, successful occasion organised by officers specifically to entertain the sisters. Elsie noted in her diary that 'The dance began at 8.45, it was splendid. I didn't dance at all but enjoyed watching them all the same.'

Elsie's reluctance to dance was partly due to tiredness and partly because she had so many suitors. Several officers made a beeline for her as soon as she arrived, cajoling and urging her to dance. Not wanting to show favouritism, Elsie decided that she would not dance with any of them. She did, however, take a shine to a young officer named Edmund. He did not pester her to dance but simply sat with her for a time. They exchanged information about their backgrounds, their work and their hopes for the future. Later Elsie confided to her diary, 'I like him rather, he is so nice and shy.'

Edmund was recovering from a wounded arm and was near the end of his convalescent period. Due to rejoin his regiment the following day, he asked if he could write to Elsie. Elsie consented, wistfully acknowledging that she would probably never see him again. It seemed to be the way in this wretched war, she thought. When people got close to each other, they were usually brutally torn apart again. Yet despite these awful circumstances, Elsie made a resolution there and then that she would not allow herself to become cynical or despondent. She would not let the war grind her down and crush her spirit.

Lily, Cynthia, Daisy and Emma were also making resolutions. Lily promised not to read so many romance novels. Instead, she would get out in the fresh air more often, regardless of the weather. Cynthia resolved to be more sociable, and Daisy decided that she would be more devout. Emma just wanted to devote all her spare time to her artwork.

Sat at her office desk checking the duty rotas, Matron was making a resolution to be more tolerant of Templeton's animosity. Simultaneously, however, she prayed earnestly for the return of her beloved Chitty. Trimble, meanwhile, who always approached problems with a certain degree of optimism, started the New Year by prioritising a number of issues. Thus he set about trying to resolve fuel shortages and to replace Templeton. His first January report, dated 3 January 1917, stated:

I am glad to say that the position of stress caused by the absolute stoppage of the supply of coal is rather easier, but I have not been able yet to get sufficient to allow fires in the wards; however I hear from the supply depot that in a few days they will be in a position to issue an increased quantity of coal and coke.

His later report to Lord Ranfurly, dated 24 January 1917, reveals that relationships between Templeton and Matron had reached a crisis point:

On Thursday the 19th I wrote to you with regard to Miss Chittock replacing Miss Templeton as assistant matron. Up to now I have not received any sanction but as the matter is of urgent importance to the hospital I took on myself the responsibility of securing Miss Chittocks' services.

It was normal practice to await sanction from St John's Gate in London before making any major staff changes. In this instance, however, the matter was considered to be of such a serious nature that sanction was bypassed. Thus on Friday 9 February 'Templeton, the assistant matron left the hospital on the termination of her engagement'. Staff usually left the hospital on termination of their contracts. Templeton, therefore, was an exception, and obviously left the hospital under a cloud.

A few days later, on Monday 12 February, Matron's prayers were answered when Mabel Chittock arrived at St John's to resume her earlier position as assistant matron. Members of the nursing staff gave her a tremendous welcome and heaved a collective sigh of relief. No longer buffeted about between two opposing forces, they were once again all pulling in the same direction.

For most of January and February, hospital water pipes were frozen. There was also a problem with the large disinfector because boiler tubes had burst. A new part was sent from London and Private. Cherry, the blacksmith, repaired the disinfector just in time for the next big intake of patients, over 90 per cent of whom were suffering from medical conditions and in an extremely bad way. Most were suffering from trench foot or acute bronchial infections. Major Houston from the bacteriology department, already working flat out, was asked to undertake further work relating to cerebral spinal fever. Swabs were taken from throats and noses of all contacts of patients suffering from this condition and examined in the laboratory.

Staff sickness continued to rise sharply, and Head Surgeon Major Hope was once again admitted to the officers' ward, this time suffering from a severe cold and chilblains. Trimble was very concerned:

He has not been well for some time. When he is sufficiently recovered I intend to send him down to Michelham convalescent home at Capmartin in the south of France for three weeks, and I am quite convinced that this will restore him to his normal condition of health.

Capmartin took the bulk of staff convalescent cases, most of whom simply needed a period of rest following the relentless pressure of heavy work. Sister Kane, for example, who spent a few weeks at Capmartin with her rheumatism, made a full recovery and was back at work by 18 February.

Trimble always ensured that his staff were well cared for. He also believed that sisters needed to receive some kind of monetary reward for their extra hard work during the Somme offensive: 'I believe that our nursing sisters should be given a belated Xmas present of one week's salary and a special bonus for these ladies for the year of 1916.' In addition to these monetary awards, Trimble advocated more leave for nurses to bring them in line with other military nurses working within the Queen Alexandra's Imperial Military Nursing Service (QAs). The latter received two weeks' leave every six months, but St John's nurses were only given one week's leave every six months. Although if there were special circumstances, such as a family illness, a nurse's leave could be extended by a few days. However, members of the Order at St John's Gate did point out that nurses had signed contracts that clearly stated their leave periods. They had accepted the terms and conditions of employment and these remained unchanged.

By the end of February over 45 per cent of hospital staff were off sick. Moreover, Trimble was forced to resolve yet another staff personality clash, this time in the hospital kitchen, where a new junior chef was making his mark by throwing crockery around at random. Trimble reported on 28 February:

> I very much regret to report that I do not think that Chef Wyniger who was sent here three weeks ago can remain. He and Bertone the senior chef get on very badly as Bertone says he is not a good cook; and his staying here would undoubtedly raise difficulty and unpleasantness amongst the kitchen staff.

Chef Wyniger was instantly dismissed but given three weeks' wages to help him on his way. On the same day 240 patients were admitted, three of whom died soon after arrival.

Another patient died from tetanus. At the beginning of March many nursing sisters were placed in quarantine, some suffering from German measles and others from severe septic throat infections. Lily and Cynthia were among those admitted to number twenty-four general hospital with German measles. Lily wrote to her sister Agnes:

> I don't mind the beastly rash, or being confined to bed. It's the horrible throbbing head which makes me feel simply awful, I can't even raise my head from the pillow without pain. Sister Harman is in the next bed and she says that nurses are dropping off sick like nine pins.

Elsie, meanwhile, was happily ensconced on the officer ward and still fighting off male attention:

> I had my tea in Etaples and came back to find Colonel Bicket in the ward. He was very amusing indeed. He also bought me a lovely box of chocolates, real beauties.
>
> The next day I had another invitation from Colonel Bicket, I am delighted.
>
> I had to relieve another ward this morning as there are so many sick. It is rather a muddle as no one seems to be quite sure how much they are responsible for.
>
> We took in eight new patients in the night. They are none of them so very sick, but they look pretty tired and worn out for all that.
>
> I heard the story for the first time about the Portugese officer, poor boy. Apparently, on the night of Jaunary 16th at about 9pm the interpreter to the Portugese troops informed our C.O. that a Portugese officer had accidently shot himself through the head and died of his wounds. Eleven of our officers and six non-commissioned officers were detailed to guard his body through the night. Of course, nobody really believes it was an accident.

Incidents of officers taking their own lives increased during
1916 and 1917, but they were usually hushed up to avoid scandal,
although stories of such cases inevitably filtered through to the
troops and those caring for them. Elsie would always listen to
patients who were worried, disturbed or lonely and often kept
them in her prayers. Sometimes she would read them poetry.
A cousin of hers had been given a poem on admission to a
military hospital in England and had sent her a copy. It was a
poem that always seemed to cheer her darling boys:

> Poem by J Pope.
> Big boy blue
> There's the blue of the sea and the blue of the sky
> As well as the blue of a feminine eye.
> But none of these kindle a thrill so acute
> As the elegant blue of a hospital suit.
> It's a soul stirring symbol of valour and pain
> It tells what its wearers can never explain.
> Yes what has been done and what's left to do
> Is silently preached by the Tommies in blue.
> We see them ensconced in a small running car
> And good looking kindly faced fellows they are.
> Maimed, bandaged, scarred but enjoying the ride
> The flotsam tossed up by wars merciless tide.
> Though the praise at our hearts is not taudy or faint
> We suffer from British self-conscious restraint.
> Yet I know of one hand that would like to salute
> Each gallant boy blue in his hospital suit.

Elsie never tired of reading this poem and never tired of listening
to her patients. In off-duty periods she frequently relaxed by
cycling to the beach or taking tea with one of her admirers.
But there was a subtle change in Elsie these days. Letters which
arrived from Edmund at the front struck a chord with her caring
nature. Shy, reticent Edmund was much more forthcoming in

letters than he had been at their first meeting. He wrote of Elsie's beauty, of her elegance and grace. He described the misery of the trenches and how memories of her smile lifted him when he was feeling low. Censorship laws prevented him from telling Elsie of his whereabouts, but he did his best to convey his thoughts and describe his surroundings. He described how his soldiers chased and killed rats, and how they gathered shrapnel pieces as souvenirs. He wrote of a desolate landscape ravaged by war, littered with empty water bottles, broken weaponry, scraps of clothing, human bones picked clean by birds of prey, unused hand grenades, spent cartridges and discarded bullet-peppered helmets. He told of shell holes full of freezing water, of a ghostly horizon interlaced with endless stretches of barbed wire and fields full of blood and skeletons. He described his food, stating that they sometimes ate a tasteless preserve referred to as JUO (jam of unknown origin). They also ate a substance that looked as though it ought to be honey but was completely tasteless; the Tommies called this substance golden glue. He also wrote enthusiastically of the humour and camaraderie of his men. Line by line, Edmund brought Elsie into his world, and her affection for him strengthened with each letter he sent. Often she would not receive mail for some days, and then half a dozen letters would arrive all at once.

Elsie knew how important letters were between loved ones. Writing letters home on behalf of soldiers was considered to be a vital nursing task. Whenever there was a lull in work routines, nurses would sit at a patient's bedside and write letters to his nearest and dearest. They would usually begin with 'You mustn't worry my girlie but I'm a bit under the weather', 'Hello my girlie', 'My old girl' or perhaps 'My darling'. Edmund's letters to Elsie began 'My dearest'; Elsie's letters to Edmund at this stage were slightly more formal, and she addressed him as 'Dear'. Over the coming months, however, these exchanges quickly progressed to 'My love'. Elsie kept her romantic attachment a secret for a long time: she did not want to prompt idle gossip and wanted to be sure of her feelings before she declared them to all and sundry.

On the 14 March, Elsie became ill with an infected throat and was placed in quarantine along with the rest of her ward. Elsie, a sociable creature, hated the isolation of quarantine:

> Sunday March 25th
>   My Birthday.
>   It began with the clocks being put on an hour and all unprepared for. Then the convoy prevented the men from getting their baths. We are still in quarantine and three more go out today, leaving only five. Then as Mr Wilson wasn't feeling well I went for a solitary bike ride.
>   Got reprimanded by matron for not being in bed, only ten minutes after the time, which left me wondering if she knew just what this continued isolation means, or if matrons were ever human.

Elsie remained in quarantine for a further seven days and celebrated her release by going for a long cycle ride and taking tea with the padre. Throat infections were successfully contained by quarantine procedures, but nurses were still prone to catching German measles. Trimble reported all these comings and goings of medical and nursing staff with an air of resignation. However, with his usual optimism he was looking forward to the summer and asked staff at St John's Gate to send him ten dozen Begonia bulbs. He knew more than most the horrors of the battlefields and believed that his patients needed to have a dramatically different view, a taste of beauty and serenity, in order to recover. Hospital grounds, therefore, needed to be attractive, with an abundance of brightly coloured flowers, fast-growing shrubs and lush green lawns, all designed to make patients feel as though they were a million miles away from blood-bloated rats, lice-infested clothes, stench-filled trenches and the battle-churned fields of no-man's-land.

17

In addition to sprucing up hospital gardens for the benefit of his patients and staff, Colonel Trimble introduced a series of lectures to educate them. These included French lessons and informative talks about Britain's allies. The former were well attended by convalescent patients and off-duty staff, but the latter proved to be an exercise in futility. Matron wrote an amusing letter to her sister Molly about Trimble's intellectual efforts, and this correspondence reveals that, despite Elsie's reservations to the contrary, Matron Todd was indeed human.

Yesterday at 3pm there was a lecture in the patients' mess on Belgians and the Belgian army. I had a note from the Padre asking me to let everyone know, why couldn't the lazy thing go round himself? It was a lovely evening and all the wards terribly busy so did not expect many, but it was rather a shock when I walked in with me behind the Colonel and the Padre at five past five to see just three patients sitting there, not one stretcher and no staff. The colonel turned on me as if it were my fault and I said he would never get staff to sit and listen to a lecture at five pm on a lovely evening after being all day on the wards.

Then he roared for the Sergeant Major who was nowhere to be found, but Sergeant Baron (the little one) stepped forward and said, 'I've been to every ward Sir and told them. I've eard [sic] all the sisters ask the up patients to go, but they say they know as much as they want to about Belgium and the Belgians and they don't want to ear [sic] any thinks about them and aren't coming.'

I nearly laughed aloud it was so funny and really I think the parson is the most helpless thing I ever saw! I said I'd go and find some and set off first to the mess and then dragged some unwilling patients from the wards where I met the Colonel in a fury saying he had put it off and told the man there was no one to listen to him. I said I'd just collected an audience and was going to L when the other men told me there were a lot of up patients, parson came to me and said there were now thirty in the room; so then Colonel Trimble said he should go round and say all the up patients were to come from the surgical side and there was quite a big audience, but the man was not up to very much – I don't think the experiment will be repeated.

Matron was correct. No further lectures were given on the subject of allies. New training sessions were introduced, however, on the subject of chemical warfare and gas masks. Matron noted:

An order has been received that all officers (I suppose as the dears are more precious) and fifteen per cent of the rest of the staff are to go to the gas chambers to be instructed in the use of gas masks etc. – as I suppose only fifteen per cent are to be supplied by them. I can't see it is much use. (Sisters) Church, Irwin, and self will go that we may show the others and then five sisters and four V.A.D.s

I am wondering whether to go to bed, for if the lights go out, it is such a chilly performance to dress again.

By this stage nearly all members of the nursing staff went to sleep fully clothed, partly because of the cold weather and partly because they may be needed to work during the night without prior notice. Rising staff sickness levels had also prompted a new recruitment phase, and on 28 March a new batch of VADs arrived. Among them was a lady named Elizabeth Veronica Nisbet, who liked to be called Veronica. Witty, flirtatious, pretty and gregarious, Veronica quickly made an impact with staff and patients alike. With elegant, angular facial features, light brown, shoulder-length straight hair and large, deep-set brown eyes, she was an attractive addition to the nursing team. She was also a very talented artist and frequently exchanged paintings and drawings with Emma. But whilst Emma painted serious and devout pictures, Veronica excelled at satirical drawings. Often these would parody members of staff or emphasise the friendly but competitive banter that existed between nursing members of the Order of St John and their counterparts within the British Red Cross Society.*

Veronica also parodied herself. One coloured drawing shows Veronica in a deep white bath with other nurses queuing impatiently at the bathroom door. Her caption reads, 'Possession is nine tenths of the law.' Another portrays Veronica sitting upright in her bed smoking a cigarette, with various items around her. The caption to this drawing reads 'Veronica of the lily white hands hurls defiance at the weather'. Such fresh, satirical humour was much appreciated by those who were tired, sick or simply worn out with war work.

In early April the hospital evacuated as many of its patients as possible in readiness for the next big push, and Colonel Carr instructed Trimble to turn yet another hospital ward into accommodation for officer patients. As Easter approached, the hospital was preparing to evacuate 530 patients in other ranks and fifty patients in the officer class. Easter Sunday was celebrated on the 8 April with joyous Christian services and sacred music. Hospital staff also staged a musical concert for the patients on Easter Monday. Elsewhere on the Western Front, Easter Monday signalled a new offensive at Arras. The British attack was supported by twenty-five squadrons of the Royal Flying Corps. Two hundred and eleven British aircrew had died by the

---

*   Paintings by Emma Mieville and an album containing the drawings of Veronica Nesbit are held at the Museum of the Order of St John of Jerusalem, St John's Gate, Clerkenwell, London.

end of April. Thousands of ground troops were also killed or severely injured. On the 11 April St John's evacuated 437 other ranks and fifteen officers; they admitted 595 patients on the same day. Furthermore, although the Battle of Arras petered out on 16 May, casualty numbers remained high for weeks to come.

Once again the hospital was working under extreme pressure, and nurses were quite alarmed when their seemingly invincible matron injured her foot as admissions came pouring through the corridors. She had unwittingly stood on a sharp nail, which penetrated the sole of her foot. The foot became very inflamed, so she was laid up for a few days. Fortunately, her wound healed quickly, and she was back at work within a fortnight.

By the end of April admissions to St John's numbered 2,080: 631 more cases than during the first month of the Somme fighting. Moreover, according to Trimble, the men's wounds were the worst he had ever witnessed. His reports were grim:

> Hospital working under pressure, all leave postponed.
>
> Cases we are getting are exceedingly grave. My impression is that the nature of the wounds in this last attack are generally speaking of a far more severe character than those we received after the attack of July last. Two of the officers should have gone on leave, but owing to the increased activity of the hospital I have had to cancel this.
>
> Two officers died: Second Lieut. K.H. Williamson, 7th Battalion Kings Royal Rifles and Second Lieut. B.L.M. Apperley, 6th Royal West Kents. I personally attended the funerals of these officers.

Trimble also recorded that extra work was continuing to take its toll on staff health:

> V.A.D. nurse Spafford was vomiting lots of blood and sent to Villa Tino. She was found to be suffering from a gastric ulcer. Mother was wired and is now coming over here and

able to visit her every day. I am very glad I can tell you this, as it would have been rather a dreadful thing if this girl had died whilst serving with this hospital.

I sent Sister Peter home on sick leave. This girl has not been very well for a while and I thought it better that she go home and perhaps save her from breaking down.

Yet amid the increased workloads and the switch back from medical to primarily surgical cases once more, nurses still found time for relaxation and romance. Elsie managed to meet up with Edmund on several occasions whilst he was on leave. They shared intimate trysts in little tea shops and cycle rides to Paris Plage. Elsie confided to her diary on 20 May: 'Picnicked with Edmund all afternoon. We didn't want to go to dinner so we loitered on, and finally a thunderstorm came on. It was a beautiful day and I thoroughly enjoyed it.' On 24 May, Elsie and Edmund became engaged to be married. Elsie was slightly apprehensive, writing, 'I do trust that all will be well in spite of the speed. I feel it will somehow.'

Romance was also in the air for Lily. As part of her resolution to avoid novels and embrace an outdoor lifestyle she had taken to cycling as often as she was able. On one occasion whilst cycling leisurely along a tranquil leafy lane, sheltered by poplar trees, her bicycle wobbled and veered off into a hedge. Her front tyre was punctured. Sitting down for a time under a leaf-laden beech tree, she took in her surroundings. Butterflies flitted about the hedgerows and birds darted in and out of leafy undergrowth. She was just wondering how long it might take to push her bicycle back to St John's when a kindly male voice interrupted her thoughts. A tall, athletic-looking man with a trim black, waxed moustache and thick black hair was looking down at her. He offered his hand to help her on to her feet and introduced himself as Lieutenant Andrew Haines of the Rifle Brigade. He was unable to offer her anything in the way of transport, but he did offer to push her bicycle for her. For Lily, his presence was the equivalent of a knight in shining armour. She would not, under normal circumstances, converse with strange men. However, given her dilemma and the fact that pushing a punctured bicycle a long way was quite an awkward thing to do, she accepted his offer with good grace. As they walked they began to talk of their families and work. Andrew was quite knowledgeable about wildlife and plants, and he pointed out several songbirds en route. Lily found that she was genuinely interested in his conversation.

Once they reached St John's, Andrew asked Lily to take tea with him at the earliest opportunity, and she shyly agreed. Excitement tinged with stomach-wrenching nervousness overwhelmed Lily as she reached the comfort of her bed. Later in the evening she asked Cynthia to be her chaperone for their first proper meeting. Cynthia enthusiastically agreed, but she pointed out that since they had already spent a good deal of time together walking in the woods, providing a chaperone now seemed rather pointless. Lily smiled at her friend, before firmly stating that everything in a courtship needed to be carried out in a proper manner. Etiquette could not be ignored. Cynthia simply nodded.

Two weeks later Andrew, Lily and Cynthia set out at 2 p.m. for Boulogne by train. Lily thought it rather a long way to go for a cup of tea, but Andrew was most insistent, stating with some authority that the best tea shops with the most variety of cakes could only be found in Boulogne. It was a gloriously sunny afternoon, and Boulogne was teaming with crowds of animated people. American soldiers, who were quickly nicknamed 'doughboys', had just arrived in France, and locals were greeting them with flags, flowers, food and drink. America had entered the war on the side of the Allies on 6 April 1917, but the first cohort of American soldiers and civilians had only recently arrived in Boulogne. This group contained 190 Americans. By the end of June, however, over 14,000 American troops had descended on France. Despite these new arrivals, Andrew managed to guide Lily and Cynthia to a beautiful tea shop with rather simple, rustic decorations. Posies of wild flowers adorned old wooden tables and an old oak cabinet. Wobbly wooden chairs were decorated with small embroidered cushions, and large impressionist-style paintings of farms dominated the walls. Heavy wooden-beamed ceilings were home to strings of garlic and onions, which hung precariously on metal ceiling hooks. Lily, too nervous to eat very much, looked briefly at the cakes on offer. She chose a pastry made with strawberry jam and, despite her nerves, was impressed by the taste. The pastry was light and melted in the mouth, and the jam actually tasted of strawberries. Cynthia chose a chocolate-covered cake and was equally impressed by its quality. Andrew explained that although the surroundings were quite sparse, the food was scrumptious and served with real tea or coffee, both imported from London. Lily asked Andrew why the place was teaming with Americans all of a sudden, so he talked at length about America's entry to the war. American public opinion had been swayed in favour of the Allies following the sinking of the passenger ship *Lusitania*. Sometime later, British intelligence officers had intercepted what became known as the Zimmermann Telegram, in which Germany proposed a military alliance with Mexico should America enter the European conflict. Along with German attacks on American merchant ships, this telegram also encouraged American support for the Allies. He also spoke of American Commander John Pershing, who, according to Andrew, had his work cut out training men who really did not have the first idea about soldiering. American support for the Allies, however, had convinced many that the war would soon end. Lily confessed that she knew little of politics, but she spoke to her date with some passion about the suffering she had witnessed. Lily had heard too many rumours claiming that peace was in the offing. She would not believe anything until it was certain. Cynthia, who was listening avidly to their conversation, nodded in sympathy with Lily. They both

worked at the front line of suffering and did not think much
of politicians. Andrew conceded that sometimes things had not
gone well for British forces, but he was nonetheless convinced
that politics would be a force for peace.

In his officers' mess, American neurosurgeon Harvey Cushing
was also dwelling on political issues. He had just watched a
French man, frustrated with Allied progress to date, let loose a
barrage of abuse towards his comrades. Cushing confessed to
his diary that such displays of anger were extremely unsettling.
Reflecting on the fighting nature of allies, he wrote:

> Italy all through. The Portugese a terrible lot – worse than
> useless. The only glimmer of hope is that Russia is not entirely
> eliminated and that Brussilof will put on a show in July.
>
> The Frenchman of course a brave fellow – gets worked
> up to a flame heat for a few moments and is irritable; but
> the flame soon goes out and it takes an exceptional man to
> kindle it again.
>
> British soldiers never flame – only a steady glow all the
> time – indeed it's up to the English to finish the job alone
> – with the possible help, in time, of America. We shall see.
> Disconcerted by all this, I was glad to escape to bed. Of
> course he was just letting off steam; but the first principle for
> allies is to keep the lid on.

Following a particularly trying period, staff in all base hospitals
began to reflect on the changing nature of allies and of
weaponry. They already knew how to treat patients suffering
from gunshot wounds, gas gangrene, neurasthenia, soldiers'
heart and phosgene attacks and a myriad of other complicated
surgical and medical conditions. By the end of June 1917 all staff
were trained in how to use gas mask, but these were about to
be rendered useless: Germany was about to unleash a new and
far more deadly biological weapon.

18

In early July a number of staff members were hastily given the leave they had earlier been denied. Major Hope, Major Houston, Lily, Elsie and Jane Bemrose could all be found, therefore, relaxing and enjoying the English sunshine. They took part in leisurely strolls along sunlit riverbanks and enjoyed gentle punting on tranquil lakes and lazy picnics in country woodland. Indeed, they were surrounded by picturesque, quintessential scenes of a typical English summer. There were cricket matches on village greens, croquet on garden lawns and church fetes serving time-honoured mixes of cream teas, Morris dancing, competitions and games – scenes that were a world away from artillery fire, gas gangrene and fulminating wounds. Occasionally there were Zeppelin raids on major cities, but on the surface, there seemed to be very little in the way of change. Under the surface, however, lay a stoical nation, collectively grieving for a lost generation. Almost every family had suffered bereavement.

Majors Hope and Houston spent time in their country houses with their respective families. They watched cricket, read newspapers, caught up with family gossip and toured a few military hospitals to swap notes about operation techniques and wound therapies. Major Hope was particularly keen to inform fellow surgeons about new glycerine-based dressings. In England glycerine was expensive and in short supply. After making some enquiries in France, however, Major Hope managed to buy a six-month supply of glycerine in Boulogne for £42, out of Brigade Hospital funds. As Trimble noted:

Glycerine is now being used in considerable quantities for making glycerine idoform emulsion. This preparation is giving very satisfactory results in the dressing of wounds. Major Hope is very anxious to carry out this form of treatment and I felt it was only right, in the interests of patients in the surgical side to give him every assistance.

Major Houston was also busy exchanging medical information with colleagues working in Britain. His research work on bacteriological conditions had been published and well received. But Houston was eager to expand this work to incorporate a large team of bacteriologists. He therefore encouraged colleagues to contribute their own research findings to the growing literature on cerebrospinal conditions.

Elsie, meanwhile, was spending her leave with Edmund. Matron Todd, yet again demonstrating a kindly nature underneath her brusque exterior, had extended Elsie's leave by three days to fit in with Edmund's time off. The couple enjoyed romantic walks in Richmond Park, did some shopping in Golders Green and picnicked in pretty terraced gardens near Kew. Edmund bought Elsie a beautiful ruby and diamond cluster engagement ring, and they made arrangements to marry in December. They spent some of their time visiting relatives and eventually said their fond farewells at London's Charing Cross station, both promising to write and meet up again as soon as possible. Elsie was elated and stared almost disbelievingly at her ring. This would need to be kept somewhere very safe, because nurses were not allowed to wear jewellery.

Jane Bemrose spent her vacation in Somerset near the rolling Mendip Hills. She needed to take care of her frail mother who was suffering from severe arthritis, and she had taken her to visit relatives. Jane worried considerably about her because apart from her dependable neighbours, Jane's mother had no other support. Fortunately, there was still time for relaxation. Jane spent time reading in the garden, which backed on to an orchard. From there she could see beautiful sunsets, fields of corn and green hills. Food was scarce due to battles at sea, but she made some fruit preserves and homemade bread and cycled down narrow lanes to nearby farms to collect freshly laid eggs. This was a country idyll, and for a brief, peaceful interlude she forgot the ravages of war.

Lily had managed to get some time off with her sister, Agnes. They decided that they would spend their leave on holiday in Devon with their parents. There was still no word from their brother William, and everyone was getting concerned. Stretcher-bearers were notoriously difficult to contact, and they had precious little time to write. Still, they had not heard from him for ten months, and they feared the worst. Lily and Agnes, however, tried to reassure their parents and encouraged them to stroll along the seafront every day. Their parents had inherited a cottage in Shaldon from Lily's maternal grandparents, and they loved nothing more than climbing across clifftops to admire the stunning views. This was a summer of ninety-nine ice creams, boat rides across the mouth of the River Teign and bracing walks along the seafront. Lily felt as though in a dream. Although coastal defences were visible, there were no sounds of rumbling artillery, no grating din of surgeons sawing as limbs were being amputated, no early morning wake-up calls, no queues for the bathroom and nobody shouting 'put out that light'. Instead, she was lulled to sleep by sounds of gentle waves lapping on the shore and seagulls calling across the bay. In the morning she could open her bedroom window and breathe fresh air. There was no reveille, no cold enamel basin and no rushing to get dressed for duty. She wrote a long letter to Andrew, describing the sights and sounds of her environment. She felt as if she were in a place suspended in time, surrounded by a bubble of contentment. She knew the bubble would soon burst, and then she would be back on the wards with red chapped hands and blistered, aching feet. But for a time at least she was blissfully reminded of the world's beauty.

Back in Étaples, Trimble was also admiring beauty. His plans for the hospital gardens had come to fruition, and a profusion of colour swept across the hospital centre ground. The ten dozen begonias supplied by the Order cast a carpet of red and deep orange along neatly trimmed borders. Purple and lilac coloured Virginia stock grew next to green shrubs, scenting the air, along with red, cream, pink and yellow roses. Purple and pink sweet peas had been persuaded by green-fingered orderlies to grow up wooden trellises along the gangways to wards, and verdant green lawns had been mowed to perfection. Trimble and his men had created an oasis of peace that resembled, as much as possible, an English country garden.

Trimble was particularly pleased, because his garden was finished in time for a royal visit. Her Majesty Queen Mary visited the hospital on 6 July. She was shown around by Lord Ranfurly, Sir Arthur Sloggett, Colonel Trimble and Matron Todd. The queen visited all departments and spoke with surgical and medical patients. She stayed for lunch, and on leaving, turned to the commanding officer and said, 'Colonel Trimble you have a most beautiful hospital.'

Staff members were thrilled and honoured by the royal visit, with the exception perhaps of Harvey Cushing, who thought the queen to be standoffish. His view was corrected by General Sloggett, Cushing recalled:

He described his recent tour with the Queen and her party – very enjoyable – they like people to be like people. He says she is shy so I retract what I said about her stiffness.

They took all their meals together like ordinary folk. 'Mary' was very much gratified with the reception given her everywhere by the French people. Sir Arthur adds that the prince is a 'little brick' – 'dear boy' – alert, interesting and lovable – wants to get into the trenches with the others. 'Why not?' says he. 'I have plenty of brothers.' They evidently struck up a warm friendship.

The royal visit of base hospitals was a huge success and a welcome boost to morale. However, a mere six days after the queen's visit, British troops were rocked by a new chemical agent. On the night of 12–13 July Germans bombarded the Ypres salient with 50,000 mustard gas shells. There were 3,000 casualties on this occasion, and on 21 July, when the gas was used again, there were 4,000 casualties. Mustard gas quickly became the most feared of all chemical weapons. When released into the trenches the gas was a faint yellow colour, which insidiously seeped through clothing, blistering skin and lungs.

Mustard gas was so called because it released a strong pungent smell of mustard oil.* The gas stayed on the ground a long time after its release, and anyone touching the skin or clothing of a contaminated person also became contaminated. Some victims of mustard gas initially displayed very little in the way of symptoms but later died of blistered lungs and enlarged hearts. It was not unusual for men to die two or three weeks after contamination. Victims usually suffered from swelling of their throats and lungs, and a distinctive widespread rash of tiny purple bruises. Larger patches of purple bruising were also visible in areas where clothing may have been tighter such as around soldiers' waistbands. Gas masks were useless against this chemical agent because it was absorbed through the skin.

It was extremely distressing to nurse terminal victims of mustard gas. Lily wrote to her sister in late July:

It is truly frightful to see such tall, muscular men fighting for every breath. Blue in the face they gasp and foam.

---

* It took the British a year to produce its own version of mustard gas. It was made at Avonmouth near Bristol and the substance was so lethal that nearly 70 per cent of the workforce involved in mustard gas production became severely ill. Seven people died in the factory in as many months because safety precautions were inadequate. As late as 2013, chemical experts from Porton Down were required to examine the site for contamination risks before a new factory could be built on the same site.

Frothy white bubbling mucous pouring from their mouths
and noses. We pray for their release from suffering – there is
nothing else we can do.

If soldiers were able to gain access to medical attention soon
after a gas attack, then oxygen therapy worked well on the
majority of victims. A third of these victims were evacuated
to England, with two thirds remaining at base hospitals or
convalescent homes in France. Of those who remained,
approximately 90 per cent were able to resume their duties
within a month. A return to duty, however, did not indicate
a full recovery. Almost 100 per cent of gas attack victims
continued to experience impaired lung function and chronic
bronchitis long after the war had ended.

Lily had stayed at the bedsides of gassed men who had no
hope of recovery, writing final letters to their loved ones. She
tried not to think of how recipients of such mail would react.
There was no time to dwell on sorrow. On Tuesday 31 July
another big push commenced. This time near Ypres. According
to the official war diary, convoys with large numbers of
wounded men were arriving at St John's nearly every night
and day throughout August and September. During the latter
month casualties, mostly stretcher cases with severe abdominal
wounds, came directly from Messines Ridge. Furthermore, the
presence of hostile aircraft circling around Étaples made night-
time operations almost impossible. Medical staff and nurses were
exhausted and war weary. Elsie, normally sociable and energetic,
stated in her diary, 'I'm so tired I don't think I can go out.' A few
days later at 11.30 p.m. she wrote, with some concern, 'Heard
my first bomb dropped at anything like close distance. Two
dropped on No. 11 Camiers, killed a medical officer and five of
the staff (Americans) and wounded nine patients.'

Sunny summer weather gave way to thundery downpours.
Then rain poured without respite throughout autumn. Yet
again, muddy terrain severely hampered fighting as British

troops scrambled up well-defended inclines in an attempt to seize Passchendaele. Battlegrounds were so thick with pasty, chalky mud that it took three men to prise a soldier's boots off his feet. By October fighting conditions were dreadful, with men slipping and sliding in mud, crawling on their bellies across quagmires and shell holes. Morale was waning. The Eastern Front was on the point of collapse due to the Russian revolution, and heavy losses on the Western Front had robbed many men of their fighting spirit.

19

Despite torrential rain and battlegrounds of slimy mud, Passchendaele was eventually captured by British and Canadian troops on 6 November 1917, after just over three months of heavy fighting. Allied casualties amounted to 275,000, with 70,000 dead. Wards at St John's were full and heavy, with an abundance of helpless men. German aircraft flew over base hospitals nearly every night, picked out against the darkness by the beaming, bright white glares of searchlights. Anti-aircraft guns flashed and fired at these aerial enemy intruders, whilst bombs landed in a nearby training camp. Amid smoke-filled air, and choking on dust, people gradually emerged from the debris – unscathed this time. But the growing threat of further bombardment was ever present. Night-time operations on the wounded were carried out intermittently by electric torchlight. Under these conditions it was not uncommon for operations to take twice the usual time.

Constant aerial activity also interfered with sleep patterns. Early in November Elsie became unwell. A combination of exhaustion and a sore throat had left her feeling very lethargic. She tried to shake off her malaise by going for a cycle ride, but only succeeded in rupturing two peripheral veins in her leg. She consulted Major Hope and was admitted to Villa Tino for a period of rest on 5 November. Not long after her admission, Elsie became feverish, tossing and turning in her immaculate bed. Her body temperature oscillating between extremes of hot and cold, and her bed sheets soaked with sweat, she suffered from periods of delirium and slept fitfully. It took a few days for her temperature to return to normal; she had no recollection of her delirium. She was showered with flowers, chocolates and good wishes by her friends, but her health was slow to improve.

On 16 November the dedication of the new hospital chapel was conducted by Bishop de Pencier of New Westminster British Columbia. Elsie manage to return to St John's just in time for the service, although she was not considered well enough to resume her nursing duties. She did not regain her strength and simply sat in the sisters' mess for two days quietly sewing. She looked pale and wan, but she managed to take tea with friends and the padre. With an air of resignation, Elsie left St John's and departed for England on 19 November. She promised faithfully to write to Dora Little, Jane Bemrose, Lily and Cynthia, all of whom were sad to see her go. But a somewhat frail Elsie was not downhearted: she had a December wedding to plan and a new future with Edmund to embrace.

For a brief time period, however, it looked as though Elsie's imminent wedding might be cancelled. A few days after her arrival in England, Elsie attended a medical appointment with a consulting physician named Mr Low on 22 November, with Major Hope also present. Elsie's illness was feared to be tuberculosis.

Fearing the worst, Elsie felt compelled to tell her fiancé of her illness. Edmund was emphatic – the wedding would go ahead as planned. Marriage vows included a promise to love each other in sickness and in health, and he would ensure that she was well cared for. Besides, Edmund had already had a recent health scare of his own. A victim of mustard gas, he had spent six weeks at a French chateau recuperating with other officers. It may well be, he argued, that both of them would suffer the long-term consequences of war during their married life. Relieved by his approach to their forthcoming wedding, Elsie felt happy and content. In her diaries and letters she always described her time with Edmund as 'sweet joy' and was convinced that this joy would see them through.

Back in Étaples, hasty preparations were being made to celebrate Christmas. Members of the musical stage group PUO were preparing a series of concerts and plays. A brass band, consisting mainly of officers, was rehearsing for Christmas Eve carols, and Matron was busy sorting out bran tub gifts for all of the wards. A group of orderlies with carpentry skills had made small wooden stables for each ward, complete with a crib, well-chiselled, painted statuettes of the Holy Family, carefully carved angels, shepherds with their sheep and three wise man with their gifts. Veronica and Emma had painted the stable backdrops and advised on the figurines. Each nativity scene was resplendent with a lantern-shaped star. Every sister was also supplied with a Christmas tree for their wards.

This year, courtesy of American forces, there was a consignment of beef, along with numerous boxes of paper decorations and Christmas cards. The latter, however, all had the same greeting: 'A Merry Christmas and a Happy New Year', which was the brief greeting approved by censorship rules. Lily, busy making brightly coloured paper garlands, was looking forward to seeing Andrew once more. She hadn't the foggiest idea where he was. His letters were affectionate and interesting, and he always described his surroundings, his men and sometimes even his feelings. He wrote of bully beef, of rat-catching competitions amongst the men, of practical jokes that lifted the men's spirits and of mock sports days. He wrote of a Lancashire lad who was wiry and built like a 'pull through' (a very narrow instrument used for cleaning a rifle), who told stories every evening and even wrote poetry. Some of the men made fun of him, but they listened to his words all the same. Lily's replies to Andrew were also tender, sometimes expressing her feelings of sorrow for the men in her care, other times revealing the joy of watching men as they responded to treatment. She wrote of her sister and her concern for William. On Christmas Eve she wrote:

This evening we paraded down the gangways singing carols
to the men. They do so love the singing poor chaps, even the
weakest of them try to join in. We wrapped up warm in our
big long overcoats because the northerly wind is bitterly cold.
My face was red raw and my hands frozen when I clutched
my lantern, even though I have a good supply of mittens.
Strong icy gusts of wind will probably bring snow soon.
Christmas snow is so romantic don't you think? Romance
is wonderful and I do miss you my dearest, but right now I'd
settle for a cup of cocoa.

Lily had also received a deluge of cards and letters on Christmas
Eve, some of which had taken a long time to reach their
destination. A letter from a friend named Rose in England
stated, 'We are hurtling towards Christmas and our dear boys
still look so glum. The ladies of the Committee have knitted
hundreds of bed socks. If there are any spare we nurses will stake
a claim. Nights are so very cold.'

Lily kept all her letters, tied up with different-coloured
ribbons, in a bedside draw. One day, when the war was over,
she planned to read all of them over again. Perhaps she would
even show them to her grandchildren, though future dreams of
marriage, children and grandchildren seemed a lifetime away.
But one thing she had discovered during this wretched war
was the importance of hope. It was a word on everyone's lips,
particularly on those of injured soldiers dictating letters home:
'I hope this letter finds you in the pink', 'I hope to be home
soon', 'I hope you are keeping well', 'I hope the children are
behaving' and 'I hope I will see you again in happier times'.
Hope, Lily decided, gave people the will to live.

Christmas Day 1917 was much the same as the previous
year. The morning began with prayers of thanksgiving and
with joyful religious services held in the new chapel. Then
men were encouraged to tip out the contents of Christmas
stockings on to their quilted bedcovers, revealing an

assortment of woollen scarves, hats, gloves and socks. Contents
also included pens, cigarettes, tobacco, confectionary, fruit and
nuts. These were all supplied by the Order's committee and
sent out from Halkyn House – a property in Belgrave Square
generously donated to the committee by Earl Beauchamp for
use as a supply depot. In addition to gifts and other comforts,
the depot was responsible for supplying St John's with over
71,000 dressings in 1917 alone.

Once stockings were opened and morning drinks distributed,
the singing began. Scrumptious meals were served throughout
the day, musical concerts were staged and Matron enticed some
interest in her bran tubs. Festivities were rounded off with
seasonal, alcoholic cheer whilst medical staff encouraged more
entertainment and comedy sketches. Veronica, who adored
being the centre of attention, captivated all patients with her
witty rendition of specially written poems. These made fun
of certain staff members, who were only thinly disguised in
her poetry. Some of the more mischievous orderlies had also
positioned sprigs of mistletoe in strategic places around the
hospital. Then, much to the delight of the patients, they staged
a competition to see how many unsuspecting nurses could
be lured under the mistletoe for a kiss. A dapper little orderly
named Robert Morris managed to obtain the greatest number
of kisses and was awarded a bottle of stout. This Christmas was
jollier than the previous year. A few Allied victories, however
slight, had convinced many that this time the Hun really was
on the run. Nobody wanted to tempt fate by being overly
optimistic, but there was nonetheless an almost tangible
confidence within Allied camps across the Western Front.

Christmas Day drew to a close, and Lily was getting ready
for bed. She had just put on some bed socks when a loud
knock sounded on her door. Lily opened the creaking door to
reveal a slightly inebriated orderly. To begin with he sounded
garbled, speaking so quickly that Lily could not make out his
message. When he was urged to speak slowly he managed to

inform Lily that she had a visitor – a man who he had placed on a chair outside Matron's office. Alarmed that someone was trying to visit at so late an hour, Lily grabbed her dressing gown and followed the orderly down the white-washed corridors. As she approached Matron's office, her visitor stood up. He resembled a tramp. Filthy clothes, scratched unpolished boots, face partially hidden by a grey woollen hat, the collar of his long overcoat pulled up to shelter his neck from the wind, he seemed desolate and weary. Lily was about to tell him to go away. This was not Andrew or an errant ex-patient. She took a sprightly step backwards as her visitor leaned forward. Then he quietly spoke, 'It's me Lily, it's me.' Lily, recognising his voice instantly, looked into his eyes and wept tears of joy. This was her Christmas miracle: her brother, William, standing before her, weary from travelling, caked in dirt, with his face an unshaven mess and his eyes lighting up at her recognition. Lily threw her arms around him and asked the orderly to bring brandy and food. A short while later, Lily had guided William to a bathroom and organised a makeshift bed. He was in dire need of a good, long sleep. There would be time tomorrow for him to tell Lily his story. For now, it was enough that he was safe.

First thing on Boxing Day morning Lily consulted Matron. A few officers were on leave, and within a matter of minutes a proper bed in the officers' quarters was secured for William. Some toiletries, shaving equipment and clean clothes were given to him by some of the officers and breakfast was served to him in bed. Matron, as usual, calmly took control of the situation. She was superb: she telephoned the Allied base hospital where Agnes was working and arranged for her to have some special leave. Then she gave orders that a telegram should be sent as soon as possible to Lily's parents. Finally, she placed her sitting room at Lily's disposal, and later that day William spoke of his ordeal.

He had been trying to retrieve a body from the battlefield but had only gone a few hundred yards before he was blown clean into the air. When he landed he fell forward and was unconscious for a long time. Surrounded by dead bodies, he awoke feeling sick and dizzy. His helmet was still on, but there was blood all over his face, seeping through his mouth and nose. His ears were humming and his right arm felt numb. He tried to stand up, but his head was swimming. He vomited twice and tried to crawl back to his trench. At some point he lost consciousness again. When he awoke he found himself in a hospital in Rouen. He had sustained a gunshot to his head, which was operated on successfully. Numbness in his arm had subsided, but he was left with a long period of amnesia. Apparently there were no identification papers on his body when he was discovered, and try as he might, he could remember nothing.

It was only thanks to some lengthy, detailed detective work undertaken by the British Red Cross that he was eventually identified. From that stage onwards he gradually remembered snippets of his past. Yet, even then, there were large gaps in his memory. Then one day a patient next to him was very thirsty and shouted 'Sister' very loudly. Suddenly he remembered: yes, he had sisters! Images of faces began to dance around his mind and he relayed them to an elderly Red Cross lady, who was painstakingly trying to piece together fragments of his life. This process of recall took some months and doctors remained reluctant to discharge him. By November, however, William had remembered that his sisters were nursing in France, and he was determined to find them. He was unsure of their exact whereabouts and feared they might be on leave in England. Nevertheless, with the help of Red Cross workers and some Christmas goodwill, he managed to discover that they were in Étaples and Boulogne. His commanding officer gave him special leave, so William set out to travel from Rouen to Étaples. Weather conditions had hampered the last stage of his journey and thus he had walked the last 30 miles in freezing temperatures, simply hoping to find his sisters.

Lily was astounded by her brother's story, which was recounted yet again the following day for the benefit of Agnes. William seemed to be quite recovered from his surgery and amnesia, but Lily, concerned about his health, asked Major Hope to examine William and assess his medical status. His verdict was that William needed to return home for further rest. After a week in Étaples, therefore, he travelled home to England. He did not return to active service.

Lily sighed with relief; it was good to think of William safe and well, far away from the line of fire. Later in the day Lily received a letter from Elsie with more good news: the wedding had gone ahead despite her ailments. Elsie wrote:

My Wedding Day

Got up early and packed, after a very pleasant remaining half an hour with Elizabeth [her cousin] in bed. Began to put on my glad rags about 10am and was so happy and excited. Mrs Baker [the dress maker] came and fixed up all the wreath and veil and it really looked nice. Edmund came for a while but I wasn't allowed to see him.

Mrs Baker and my bridesmaid Elizabeth (looking very sweet in a white taffeta frock) went down in a taxi at 11.30 am. Everything went well and all our friends seemed to be there. Sir Patrick Manson gave me away.

Lily folded the letter, tied it with yellow ribbon and placed it with her collection. Good things were happening. William was safe, Elsie was married and news was filtering through the hospital grapevine that British Empire forces had recaptured Jerusalem. Consoled by these recent events, she leant back on her bed and said her prayers.

20

New Year 1918 at St John's began with the arrival of sixty stretcher cases and the ominous sound of enemy aircraft droning above. Trimble, in a positive mood as usual, had recently implemented an exchange scheme between the hospital orderlies and men serving with No. 130 St John Field Ambulance Unit. This scheme lasted for a few months. During the first week of January a number of musical concerts were staged for the benefit of the patients. Then, on the 6 January, Trimble issued orders that as many staff and patients as possible needed to gather in the dining hall to listen to a new proclamation from His Majesty the King:

> To my people – The world wide-struggle for triumph of right and liberty is entering upon its last and most difficult phase. The enemy is striving by desperate assault and subtle intrigue to perpetuate the wrongs already committed and stem the tide of a free civilisation. We have yet to complete the great task to which, more than three years ago, we dedicated ourselves.
>
> At such a time I would call upon you to devote a special day to prayer that we may have the clear-sightedness and strength necessary to the victory of the cause. This victory will be gained only if we steadfastly remember the responsibility which rests upon us, and in a spirit of reverence and obedience ask the blessing of Almighty God upon our endeavours. With hearts grateful for the Divine guidance which has led us so far towards our goal, let us seek to be enlightened in our understanding and fortified in our

courage in facing the sacrifices we may yet have to make before our work is done.

I therefore hereby appoint January 6th – the first Sunday of the year – to be set aside as a special day of prayer and thanksgiving in all the churches throughout my Dominion. And require that this proclamation be read at the services held on that day.

George R.I.

The recently appointed Reverend C.H. Mylne complied with the king's wishes by holding a special service that very day. Another important service of thanksgiving was held in the hospital chapel on 11 January to mark the recapturing of Jerusalem. However, Cynthia recorded that 'Not all patients are keen on worship, and it takes quite some effort to persuade them to attend Holy Communion'.

Approximately a third of all 'up patients' did attend religious services of their own accord. The remainder were cajoled or ordered to attend chapel. Officers were more likely to demonstrate faith and an adherence to Christian principles, in part because they genuinely believed in God and also because they were required to set an example to their men. Like all members of the Order, Trimble was a steadfast Christian, an honourable man who encouraged faith-based activities. He also invited members of other hospitals to attend chapel services and to exchange entertainment programmes. In particular, he established a strong bond with the nearby Canadian hospital. They often helped each other out in times of staff shortages and gave concerts to both sets of patients. For instance, a concert was given on 29 January by Willow O'Wisps, which involved Canadian and St John's medical and nursing staff.

For the first few months of 1918 the hospital experienced the usual problems of frozen pipes and weather-related supply shortages. In March large numbers of casualties arrived from St Quentin, similar to those received the previous November and

December from Cambrai. Convoys usually arrived at night, and because of enemy aircraft, there were immense difficulties with unloading patients at this time. Étaples was severely bombed on several occasions, and in order to avoid injury, members of the population were trekking out to surrounding countryside. By April this was a nightly occurrence.

Life on the wards, however, continued much as normal. Medical and nursing standards remained high, and letters of thanks continually poured into Trimble's office. The following is an extract from an ex-surgical patient named Major Hemelryk:

> I don't think I shall ever forget all the kindnesses I received at your hands and those of Major Hope, and all those good and kind nurses.
>
> Do convey to them my most heartfelt thanks and I only wish I could adequately express on paper the gratitude I feel, not to speak of the absolute admiration. I think those nurses were simply wonderful and no praise is too high for them.
>
> Nothing was too much trouble for them, and I do not think I shall ever forget all they did for me.
>
> Please convey my warmest thanks to the matron, and if it is not insubordinate my heartiest congratulations on such a wonderful hospital where kindness has been brought to such a pitch of perfection.

On the 11 May a case of cerebrospinal meningitis was identified on Q ward, and twenty-three beds were closed until patients' contacts were located and proved to be free of infection. There were also cases of mumps, measles and tuberculosis.

By the middle of May, hospital staff were getting increasingly anxious about hostile aircraft, and with good reason. There were numerous close calls before serious air raids inflicted damage. Then, without warning, on 17 May an air raid obliterated part of the Canadian hospital situated next to St John's. The raid lasted over two hours. In total thirty-eight bombs were dropped on the Canadian hospital and the surrounding area. Fifty-nine people were killed, and ninety-nine were injured. Among the dead were eight patients, three nursing sisters and one officer. Cushing reported:

> Colonel Trimble, the jolly Irish C.O. of St Johns, had his clothes punctured by a bomb which fell close to him and some of his people received slight wounds; but the Canadians were badly hit – two hours lying on the ground with torpedoes falling and bursting about, followed by an effort to succour the wounded and collect the dead in ones' camp, it is nerve racking to say the least.

A fire alarm had sounded at St John's the moment an incendiary bomb dropped on the Canadians next door. All nurses proceeded to their wards, and Matron was met in the corridor by a strange sight, which in other, less dire, circumstances would have been very amusing. Lily, Cynthia, Veronica and Daisy were all marching along the gangways with white enamel washbasins placed firmly on their heads to protect them from shrapnel. Matron considered this to be an inspired idea. Thus nursing sisters were instructed to use similar basins to protect their helpless patients.

Writing of this dreadful night, Matron recorded:

> It was fortunate they [the nurses] did go to the wards. The next morning one sister who was in bed asleep when the first bomb fell, found a large piece of shrapnel in her pillow and the cubicle next to her bed was riddled with fragments of bombs. Many of the dying and wounded from the next hospital and the camp were brought into our wards and as it was possible to open the theatre some of them were taken there.
>
> We never heard what the total number of casualties in the area was on that night – but it must have been tremendous.

I was very much impressed with the convoy of ambulance drivers (they have a woman's convoy at Etaples). The girls were out on the road bringing in the wounded during the whole time of the raid. Our own staff and sisters, V.A.D.s and orderlies were splendid and no one showed the least panic or alarm.

British newspaper reports of this bombing were full of heroic stories:

The more serious cases had to remain in their beds till a party of St John Ambulance men arrived with stretchers. They were plucky fellows, for they had to risk their lives to get to us but they did their work well and saved hundreds of the boys.

In response to this fierce attack, Trimble ordered hundreds of sandbags; these were filled by German prisoners of war and banked up against all hospital wards, up to window ledges. Dugout shelters were constructed the next day, and orders were given for all 'up patients' to make their way to shelters in the event of an air raid. Orderlies also made a trench outside nurses' quarters for sisters and VADs. Deep shelters were also planned, but there was no time to finish them before the German bombers returned on 19 May.

German aircraft released a magnesium flare to highlight target areas, and bombing began at 10.30 p.m. Four bombs dropped within hospital grounds along with eleven others near the men's quarters. Casualties, when compared to the earlier attack on the Canadian hospital, were relatively light, with twenty-seven wounded and fourteen killed. Among the dead were Private H. Clark from Scunthorpe, aged 23; Private R.C. Bell of Bristol, also aged 23; Lieutenant/Corporal McConway from Jarrow, 25; and Corporal/Acting Sergeant Pickett, attached from the Northumberland Fusiliers.

Lily was horrified by this sequence of events. Every hospital had a large red cross painted on the roof, clearly indicating that occupants were in the business of saving lives rather than taking them. She had overheard officers arguing outside the dining hall, some stating that German bombers were really attempting to blow up nearby railway lines and bridges, and hospitals were simply collateral damage. Later that week, however, came a report that one bomb was dropped on a hospital smack bang in the middle of a clearly visible red cross. Lily did not give the enemy the benefit of doubt. As far as she was concerned, there were no excuses. Even Dora Little, who was always prepared to forgive anybody anything, was beginning to lose patience.

Cushing also expressed doubts about German bombing strategy:

> No damage of military significance was done, or could have been done, except confusion of the area. This may be their intent. If it is, and they come again tonight, the demoralization will certainly be complete. The time before, everyone thought they were after the railroad and excused them; the second time the bridge across the Canche a mile or so further on; but this time what?

Matron too was tiring of the incessant raids:

> The weather just then was most thundery and oppressive, and those few days were most trying. On Monday they left us in peace. But on Tuesday we had them over again and very frequently – almost every other night after that. It was so bad for the patients, especially the helpless ones that we evacuated all we possibly could to England. On the night of Thursday 30th Corpus Christi, they refrained from bombing any of the hospitals but did terrible damage in Etaples, killing a great number of French civilians. (There was a complete exodus of all inhabitants the next morning.)… After Thursday we

felt comparatively safe, and said, well they will not bomb the
hospital now.

Other members of staff shared Matron's opinion. Considerable
damage and havoc had already been wreaked on all base
hospitals; it hardly seemed worthwhile for German bombers
to return. Lily hoped they were right. Trying to grab clothes and
dress in the middle of the night, when huts were shuddering
and shelves were falling off the walls, was no easy task. Bombs
falling made a tremendous, earth-shattering noise, bursting
eardrums and smashing glass to smithereens. Some people were
now a bag of nerves, and it had taken Lily some time to regain
composure. Cynthia was finding sleep difficult, waking every
few minutes thinking she could hear hostile aircraft. Daisy had
gone off her food, which was a worry considering she was
already so thin and dainty. Veronica, however, was in defiant
mood, hoping to come face-to-face with a German, to give
him a piece of her mind. Meanwhile, Lily wondered whether
it was prudent to sleep with an enamel basin over her face,
eventually deciding against the idea.

   In many respects, however, Lily had surprised herself. She had
expected to crumble in the face of danger or to lose her wits
at the very least. Instead, she felt angry. Helpless patients and
kind staff members were being put through the wringer and
for what? Not one person within hospital walls could be seen
as a danger to the enemy. Yet the enemy seemed hell-bent on
bombing them. Lily did not flinch when bombs rained down,
neither did her friends and colleagues. This stoical bravery
was a constant surprise. Earlier in the war she had been full of
self-doubt, now she was self-confident. Somehow along the
way, the war had moulded her character into something rather
unexpected. For this metamorphosis alone, she would remain
forever grateful.

21

Once clearing parties had repaired the hospital bomb damage of 19 May, spring sunshine lifted the spirits of otherwise slightly jittery personnel. Hospital life returned to normal. Two-thirds of patients were evacuated to England during the following ten days in preparation for spring offensives. Then, in the early hours of 31 May a convoy arrived with 113 casualties. Ten of these were walking wounded who settled down immediately, and the remaining were stretcher cases who needed urgent attention and surgical operations. It was Lily's day off, and she was busy writing a long letter to Andrew. Veronica had gone for a cycle ride to Cecil Plage beach. Cynthia was vigorously cleaning bedside tables in one of the medical wards, and Daisy was serving barley water and lemonade to some surgical patients. Sister Jane Bemrose was occupied with dressing wounds, and Catherine Warner was preparing to administer patients' drugs. Matron and Chitty were drawing up duty rotas, whilst Trimble was inspecting dugouts and sandbag positions. Some orderlies were tending the garden, pulling up invading weeds, watering new flower shoots and trimming grass borders in the central precinct. Everyone was going about their business in a calm and disciplined fashion.

When evening descended on this ordered, tranquil hospital, officers were playing cards in their quarters; Lily and her friends were drinking cocoa, cosily huddled around Veronica's bed while she held court with her irreverent imitations of senior nursing staff; and night nurses were making their patients comfortable for sleep.

By 10.30 p.m., however, the familiar droning of enemy aircraft could be heard overhead once more. The bombers had returned. Yet again a stunningly bright magnesium flare lit up the sky, but this time all hell broke loose. Like incessant, deafening rolling claps of thunder, an avalanche of bombs dropped on St John's. Earth-shattering explosions of earthquake proportions erupted from every conceivable direction, walls shuddered and ceilings collapsed under the tremendous impact of aerial attack. Staff ran to their stations as splinters of glass and falling timber huts trapped, maimed and killed. With the earth trembling and convulsing under their feet, Lily and her friends grabbed their enamel basin helmets and scurried through shaking corridors and falling shelves towards their patients. Matron and Chitty calmly walked the length and breadth of the wards, giving words of reassurance to their patients and shouting instructions to nurses above the din of ear-splitting bomb blasts. Dora Little and Margaret Ballance were guiding up patients out of the wards when three orderlies suddenly pushed them to the ground and rolled them into nearby dugouts. Seconds later a huge explosion rocked the ground a few feet away from them. Lily and Cynthia were rushing around the medical wards, shouting at patients to take cover under their beds, when they too were shoved by orderlies in the direction of dugouts. Meanwhile, Trimble, Captain William Wilson and Captain Frederick Hall dashed about with fire extinguishers, attempting to douse roaring wildfire flames, which quickly took hold of the wooden hospital huts.

The first large bomb had dropped without warning on the centre of a medical ward (O ward). Sister Annie Bain, who was in charge of O ward on night duty, was killed instantly as she sat at her desk writing reports. Seven patients were also killed instantly. Three orderlies, Sergeant C. Young, Private J. Scott and Private I. Roberts, desperately attempted to save remaining patients but were killed outright by a second bomb. There was no time for them to run and no time to get occupants out of the ward. Lily, watching the scenes of brutal destruction from the relative safety of a dugout, was convinced that everyone who remained in the hospital must have been killed. A visibly shaken Cynthia began to pray in earnest, encouraging patients to do likewise. Loudly and insistently they all repeated the Lord's Prayer as the deluge of bombs rained down.

Sister Catherine Warner and a medical officer established a rudimentary dressing station to deal with minor wounds whilst sisters Jane Bemrose and Molly McGinnis rushed from ward to ward assessing patients' wounds and guiding some to the safety of dugouts. Molly McGinnis actually threw herself on to the bed of a helpless patient, acting as a human shield against the bombardment. Many of the up patients also assisted nurses in their endeavours to protect the helpless. Ward furniture had been blown sky high, and shards of glass peppered the whole area. Wards were demolished and operating theatre windows shattered. The ferocious bombardment continued for three hours, although Matron recalled that it felt like three days. St John's own fire brigade and orderlies bravely rescued patients from debris whilst nurses attended to the wounded. As Matron recounted:

> The more serious ones were carried onto beds which had just been swept clear of broken glass and splinters. Torniquets were hastily put on to bleeding limbs, by the lights of an electric torch, which could be turned on for a minute or two before there would be a shout of 'Put that light out they are over us again.' Morphine was given if it could be found, but every medicine cupboard was wrecked and in most of the wards the water supply had been damaged and no taps could be turned on.
>
> I wish I had time to tell you how splendid both patients and orderlies were in the way they looked after helpless patients and thought of their safety. We were accustomed to the sisters thinking only of their patients at this time, that it seemed quite strange to hear the men insisting on them 'taking shelter' under beds and wherever the aeroplanes were sighted over us.

By morning the devastation was clear for all to see. The northern end of the hospital was completely destroyed, and the remainder resembled a collapsed pack of cards. Paperwork, furniture, bedding and bedsteads littered the ground for miles around. Aside from the cardiograph department, everything lay in ruins. Staff, in a state of delayed shock, observed their surroundings disbelievingly. Matron reported:

> We were a very limp and pallid looking collection of people when it was at last daylight – enough to see each other. It was heart breaking to see our poor little hospital which we were all so proud of in such ruins.
>
> I think we were all glad that there was so much to do, so there was no time to think. As early as possible from after 8am we evacuated all remaining patients to other hospitals for the wards that were left standing were not safe.

Later that day British Red Cross ambulances arrived in Étaples to collect most of St John's nurses to take them to Boulogne. From there, they travelled to England for a period of leave. Trimble kept a skeleton staff behind to help with the sorting and packing of hospital equipment. Injured sisters Thompson, Mckinnon, Eadie, Glubb, Higginson and O'Donnell were sent to a sick sisters' hospital for treatment; along with VAD Ida Bull; the latter sisters also suffered from shell shock. Members of nursing staff who remained in Étaples spent every night at the sisters' convalescent hospital in Hardelot. These included the matron, assistant matron, sisters Bedford, Slevin, Hayden, John, Ryecroft, Worsley, Murray and Stubington, and VADs White and Trimble. Medical officers and orderlies chose to sleep in what remained of the wards. Fearful of enemy bombers, some staff from all base hospitals trekked out into the woods each evening to sleep.

A sombre Colonel Trimble sent a telegram on 1 June to Lord Ranfurly informing him of the disaster, before attempting to catch up on sleep. Cushing recorded, 'Colonel Trimble is worn out and in his bed, he deserves a V.C., having called for volunteers to help extinguish a fire in one of the wards while bombs were falling on every side.'

Trimble continued to write his reports, however, and was mightily relieved that the death toll was much smaller than at first anticipated. Fortunately, the hospital was only half full, and due to Trimble's foresight with regard to sandbagging walls, some protection had been afforded to patients. Recently dug trenches also helped to lessen casualty numbers. Without these precautions, Trimble was convinced that at least two further wards would have been blown into the air, killing all occupants. He was also proud of the way his staff had behaved during this recent crisis, informing Ranfurly:

> When the alarm was given, everybody went to their station; the prompt and good discipline carried out to my mind accounts for the small number of casualties, because the explosion of four large bombs, two between the wards, and two on the side had a terrific effect. I shall never forget it as long as I live.
>
> I have again to record the splendid heroism and devotion to duty displayed by all ranks, particularly by the sisters; I am recommending at least one of them for a military medal. This last act of Hun barbarity should cause much indignation at home, and gives ample opportunity of appealing to the public for funds to carry on the hospital.

Trimble was also gratified to realise that this latest disaster did not signal the end of St John's hospital. General Carr, Director of Medical Services in France, was eager to retain the hospital by relocating staff and equipment to Trouville. This move was organised by the Royal Engineers.

In the meantime, however, Trimble sent all officers on leave, on the condition that they could be recalled at any time.

Most were in dire need of a rest and considerably rocked by the air raid's intensity. Yet despite the obliterating devastation wreaked by German bombers, Trimble still exhibited signs of optimism, writing a reasonably upbeat report to Ranfurly on 5 June:

> Without exaggeration I think we can say we came through a form of hell, but Thank God, the calamity might have been rather worse. It is hard to believe that men and women could get so unnerved and rattled in so short a time; it is not the actual time of bombing that one feels it but afterwards.
>
> However, we are all in good heart and nearly back to our normal conditions. The work of packing up the hospital is proceeding rapidly, and the matron, assistant matron and the nursing staff who remained have done truly excellent work.
>
> I have made certain recommendations for immediate reward for my M.O.s, sisters and men of the company. I can never forget the discipline, fortitude and bravery exhibited by the entire staff of the hospital. It was splendid beyond description. I was fortunate to have command of such a brave lot of people and they were a great support to me in this very trying time.
>
> Well my Lord, the best hospital in France has been considerably shattered, yet there is sufficient life left to keep the flag of St John flying.

Trimble's spirit of optimism in the face of such adversity was infectious. He told jokes, helped with the packing of equipment and maintained a positive approach throughout the uprooting of his beloved hospital.

Air raids continued in their intensity despite the fact there was little left to bomb. On 1 July an air raid began at 12.10 a.m., lasting for one hour and a quarter. On 4 July Trimble sent the first consignment of equipment and personnel to Trouville. These included one officer and 110 other ranks. Trimble, along with his small cohort of nursing staff, arrived in Trouville on 8 July. From then on the new hospital began to take shape. Members of the nursing staff often helped out in other hospitals while St John's was being rebuilt, and their spirits were uplifted by news of Allied advances. On 8 August 1918 Allied forces began a new offensive and quickly achieved a decisive victory. The British fourth army, led by Henry Rawlinson, advanced 7 miles on the first day alone, and hundreds of German soldiers surrendered. The 8 August became known as a 'black day for the German army' and signalled the end of trench warfare. This was the start of the Allied 100-day offensive. The Second Battle of the Somme began on 21 August and was key to subsequent successful Allied advances.

According to the official war diary, Trimble, medical officers and nurses took extended leave in August and September. This gave staff a much-needed opportunity to recuperate. Lily spent most of her time in England getting to know Andrew's family in Cambridgeshire. In early September Andrew took Lily to Grantchester for a picnic. They travelled at a leisurely pace by punt along the rippling River Cam to Byron's pool, so called because Lord Byron was reputed to have favoured the spot for his swimming sessions. Sunlight filtered through leafy trees, glistening on the water below. Choosing a shady spot for their al fresco meal, Andrew, who was well aware of Lily's romantic nature, quoted Lord Byron:

> She walks in beauty, like the night
> Of cloudless climes and starry skies;
> And all that's best of dark and bright
> Meet in her aspect and her eyes:
> Thus mellowed to that tender light
> Which heaven to gaudy day denies.

Lily was enthralled, and even more so when Andrew followed Byron's poetic verse with a proposal of marriage. He fumbled awkwardly in his blazer jacket and produced an emerald engagement ring that had belonged to his grandmother. He had bought a special marriage license, and he informed Lily that they could be married within the week. Lily happily accepted his proposal but on one condition. She stated emphatically that she would only get married when the war was over and St John's hospital disbanded. Strange as it might have seemed to Andrew, Lily wanted to see things through. If she married within the week, she would have to resign from St John's at a time when they still needed experienced personnel. Andrew, however, desperately wanted to keep Lily safe. Recent events and continued bombing raids in France placed Lily in considerable danger, but he could not change her mind. Their marriage plans were therefore placed on hold.

Prior to the reopening of St John's in Trouville, Trimble was eager to train nurses in new massage treatments for orthopaedic and surgical patients. Recent research had revealed that physical massage and stimulation with electric currents improved nerve function and muscle strength in post-operative patients. Trimble, therefore, instructed Matron to enquire about massage training techniques for nursing sisters. But there were a few obstacles with regard to training, as Trimble noted on 18 September 1918:

> I heard from Miss Todd two or three days ago. It appears there is a difficulty getting hospitals to accept our girls for three months training. It seems six months is usual. However, Major Hope has written to a friend at Kings College hospital who may be able to make necessary arrangements to enable girls to get an insight into electrical apparatus connected with massage, and massage itself.
>
> If this cannot be done, then we will just have to bring Miss Drummond out here, and those of nursing staff detailed to assist the department, will take up work under her instruction.

In the event, St John's nurses still in England attended a three-month course in massage therapy. However, not everyone was a fan of this new treatment. Cushing was taken ill in the summer with an undiagnosed neurological condition and prescribed massage:

> In bed getting my sensation tested, and having a female from the sergeant's school, built like a football tackle, giving me a massage. One particular thing which consists in beating my sore and wasted extremities seems to me unnecessary. I call it the barrage – I'd much prefer to have her go over me with a tank.

Regardless of its merits or failings, massage became a new and important treatment and can be viewed in many respects as a forerunner of physiotherapy. Experienced VADs Lily, Cynthia and Daisy were all instructed in basic massage techniques, along with eight nursing sisters. They completed their training just before the reopening of St John's on 1 October 1918. Eager to practise their new skills, they returned to Trouville full of news and gossip with regard to earlier staff members. Clutching English newspapers, they were also thrilled to have some good news to share with their colleagues with regard to Allied offensives. However, just as Allied forces were making good progress on the Western Front, another more sinister battle was being lost on the medical front.

The virulent strain of influenza that had laid Major Hope so very low the previous year had mutated and returned with a vengeance. People were dying like flies, and there was nothing anyone could do. Over 20 million people died from flu during the first six months of the outbreak. On the home front, by the end of October, an average of 4,500 British people were dying from flu every week. On the Western Front mortality rates from flu were climbing rapidly every day, with weekly medical reports admitting, 'with regard to the prevailing influenza epidemic we have a serious present situation'. This particular strain of flu was also very unusual in that it targeted not the young, old or vulnerable but typically those aged between 18 and 35. It was rife, therefore, in the troops of all nations currently at war, and in all those who cared for the wounded.

22

For medical and nursing teams who had valiantly fought to save men from the ravages of war, the fact that many were now dying from of a virulent strain of influenza was a cruel twist of fate. Rows upon rows of bodies were piled up outside mortuary blocks, and casualty clearing stations became units designated for the care of flu victims. Symptoms included severe headaches, high fevers, griping stomach cramps and delirium. Previously strong, vibrant young men were brought to their knees by the virus. The onset was sudden, overpowering and completely debilitating. Within a few days influenza patients usually developed pneumonia and died. Doctors could do nothing to prevent these deaths. Nurses kept patients as comfortable as possible, administered fluids and in some instances used inhalations to ease lung congestion. Cupping was sometimes helpful. This involved the heating of glass cups containing an alcohol-soaked cotton wick. The wicks were set alight to heat the cups, which were then quickly placed on the back of the chest, held in place by suction. This process was very successful in relieving severe congestion, but recovery ultimately depended on individual immune systems.[*]

As surgical cases began to wane, medical wards were soon filled with flu victims. St John's official war diary for October reveals that both nurses and patients were succumbing to the virus nearly every day. There were attempts at quarantine, but these were unsuccessful. Other medical conditions were

---

[*] Globally over 500 million people became infected with influenza between 1918 and 1920, and 50 million people died.

also on the increase, particularly venereal disease. A blood test known as the Wasserman reaction test was introduced to diagnose the presence of syphilis. An official memo sent to all commanding officers ref 647/1/18, dated 4 November, signed by Major Sheenan on behalf of the Deputy Director of Medical Services, stated:

> Wasserman reactions can now be carried out for this area at the laboratory of St John Ambulance Brigade Hospital on Tuesdays and Fridays.
>
> Pathologists should forward 5c.c. of the blood they wish examined in small corked tubes on Monday or Thursday afternoons or evenings to the above laboratory.
>
> For purposes of reference the following particulars should be furnished with a sample of blood:
> Name, number, regiment and age of patient.
> Hospital where patient is.
> Date and hour of collection of specimen.
> Situation and character of lesions.
> Length of time the disease has existed.
> Has patient previously received specific treatment?
> If so, state particulars.
> Has a previous specimen from this patient's blood been examined?
> If so, give date and particulars.

The introduction of Wasserman reactions was a big step forward in terms of diagnosing syphilis. There was still no test for gonorrhoea, however, and treatments for both forms of venereal disease were not particularly successful. Clearly medical teams were fighting a losing battle against influenza and venereal disease, but this state of affairs was not publicised on the home front. British newspapers were preoccupied with stories of glorious Allied advances and the forthcoming prospect of an armistice.

By early November the Allies had captured 362,355 prisoners and were claiming decisive victories with the passing of each day. Everyone eagerly waited with bated breath for Germany to surrender. On 10 November Lily noted in her diary, 'Everyone is impatient. A ring on the telephone gives us all the jitters. Will this be the call that ends it all? People rush to get the newspaper even though it is already two days old! Surely the end will come soon.' The following day, to the relief of all combatants and non-combatants, an armistice was signed. Trimble wrote in his Company Orders book, 'Armistice signed between Allies and Germany at 6am to take effect from 11am today. Thank God.'

On hearing the news there was elation and pandemonium. Shouts of hurrah, some whistle and trumpet blowing, people embracing each other, hugging, laughing and kissing. This was not a time for British reserve! Nurses rushed to inform their patients of the tumultuous news. Matron opened her store of medicinal brandy and measured out small tots for everyone. Infused with relief and joy, a concert party was held in the well patients' dining room at 2.30 p.m. to celebrate the end of the war. This was the start of many celebrations. Performances of music dancing and drama were a constant source of entertainment in the coming weeks. Lily wrote delightedly to Agnes, 'Patients are trying to dress up as St George – costumes most amusing.' Cushing observed:

Thus the Great War ends at the eleventh hour on the eleventh day of eleventh month 1918; and the Kaiser awakes from his forty year dream of world domination. It's a piteous spectacle. All the Kings horses and all the Kings men couldn't put Humpty together again.

Earl Ranfurly arrived on 12 November to visit St John's and thank staff for their marvellous efforts during very trying times. Trimble spent some considerable time congratulating his staff and thanking them for all of their hard work. He sombrely informed them that over 1,000 St John members had been killed on active service. This number included stretcher-bearers and those working in casualty clearing stations. The British Army had sustained nearly 3 million casualties. It was now time for staff to remember those who had made the ultimate sacrifice and to keep them in their prayers. A series of thanksgiving services were held throughout November. There were also a number of musical concerts.

As Christmas approached, sisters and VADs were in a joyful frame of mind. They had shared a close camaraderie and experienced some truly heartbreaking times. Now they could relax and enjoy the peace. Members of the PUO drama group were rehearsing *H.M.S. Pinafore*, and No. 4 Canadian depot gave a 'Bohemian Concert Party' on 20 December.

Christmas Eve was emotional. Carols were sung in the wards as usual, but nurses were remembering their old hospital and the loss of their colleagues, in particular Annie Bain, who had loved everything about the festive season. Matron lit a special candle in her memory as sisters fought back tears. Prayers were said, and newly built nativity scenes positioned near the Christmas trees. This year, free from the fear of enemy aircraft, tree lights remained switched on. As Matron told her patients on Christmas Day, light had overcome darkness in more ways than one.

Gifts were distributed on Christmas morning amid much gaiety and laughter. Even patients still in the throes of flu attempted to be joyful. Lily worked all day and well into the evening, as did all other nurses. All of them wanted to savour every minute of this peaceful season. Trimble recorded with some satisfaction that 'Xmas day was observed with much enthusiasm and much food and games.'

Matron's traditional bran tub contained a wider variety of gifts this year, and there were no fuel shortages. When the day nurses returned to their quarters, they found that Matron had placed small parcels of chocolates on every bed. They were tied up with white ribbons and decorated with paper stars. Lily, who had not had time to open her presents earlier in the day, now took great pleasure in examining her gifts: another romantic novel from Agnes, pens and notepaper from her parents – a gentle hint, perhaps, that she needed to write to them more often, an exquisite silver cross and chain plus a book of poems from Andrew, and a miniature painting from Emma. Veronica had given everyone hand-drawn caricatures, and Daisy had distributed sugar mice amongst her friends.

On Boxing Day it was the patients' turn to entertain. All who were able took part in a fancy dress parade. Indeed, Trimble recorded an 'excellent turn out'. Some were dressed as Christmas angels, others as Father Christmas or elves. A few decided it was time to parody the Kaiser, while others chose to dress up as figures from fairy tales. In the afternoon there was a dress rehearsal for a pantomime. Concerts continued for the remainder of December, and on 1 January PUO gave a second performance of *H.M.S. Pinafore* to entertain visiting guests. A dance was also held on the same day, and everyone swapped ideas for New Year resolutions. Lily resolved to marry in spring, Cynthia decided to write children's stories, Daisy hoped to begin her nurse training in a civilian hospital and Veronica and Emma wanted to pursue artistic careers. In the sisters' mess, Jane Bemrose was looking forward to taking a country holiday, Catherine Warner was hoping to be promoted back in England and Molly McGinnis laughingly stated that she would meet and marry a rich man. Matron and Chitty simply wanted to resume their civilian careers at Guy's Hospital. All were looking to the future, and yet were terribly sad at the prospect of leaving St John's.

No patients were admitted to St John's after 15 January 1919. Trimble was organising the demobilisation of staff. In his weekly report he stated:

Matron and Mabel Chittock will travel via Boulogne on 31st. Matron-in-Chief; Dame Maud McCarthy is anxious to see all matrons before they leave France. They will travel first to Paris then to Boulogne. By the end of the present month all nursing staff will have departed. V.A.D.s White and Trimble proceeded to Cannes for three weeks sick leave (recovering from flu). Sisters will depart for England on 18th and V.A.D.s returning to England will depart on 19th.

On 13 February, SS *Endcliffe* arrived in Trouville dock to transport all of the hospital stores to Southampton. Hospital buildings were sold to Mayor Mons Le Hoc of Deauville for the sum of 250,000 francs and some of the remaining hospital huts were used to house the local population, many of whom had been bombed out of their own accommodation. Other huts were turned into wards for the treatment of children with tuberculosis. Mayor Mons Le Hoc gave the Order of St John 500 francs from his own purse as a gift to the Order, in grateful thanks for its medical service in France.

Nursing sisters had been demobilised promptly, but Trimble was also concerned that his men should be demobilised too, writing to Ranfurly:

> I am particularly anxious that all these men should return to England before I leave, or at the time I go. I hold that the Company came out to do a distinct and definite job: this has been done and their work is finished, and I think in all justice to them they should be allowed to return home.
>
> It must be remembered that these men enlisted in 1915, they were not conscripts, but loyal patriotic men who came out to do their duty. It would be a great disappointment to me if any of these men were taken and distributed elsewhere.

Apparently the demobilisation of men was somewhat slower than that of nursing sisters. However, all men were demobilised by the time St John's was disbanded on 3 March. During its time St John's admitted 36,100 men. As Trimble proudly stated:

The 3rd of March 1919 brings the curtain down on our hospital. Cognisant of excellent work it was the finest of its kind in France. The hospital was sent out under the flag of St John and built up an excellent reputation. This reputation was sustained until the end.

The Order of St John had every reason to be proud of its hospital. Not only did it provide consistently high standards of care for the sick and wounded, it was also at the cutting edge of medical research. Several articles were published, such as Houston and McLoy's paper on bacteriology and transactions when dealing with wounds, which was published in *The Lancet* on 7 October 1916. Papers that focussed on X-ray techniques and some connected with the issue of soldier's heart were also influential. Furthermore, in recognition of their immense bravery under fire, some members of the medical and nursing staff were awarded medals.

Those sisters who had participated in military nursing in the hope of gaining women's suffrage were partially rewarded when the 1918 Representation of the People Act gave limited voting rights to women. In 1919, spurred on by the nation's poor health and the influenza pandemic, a Ministry of Health was established. In the same year the Nurse Registration Act was passed. However, nurses, still arguing about status, failed to agree on a professional direction. Therefore the government established a General Nursing Council (GNC). Registration for general nursing entailed a three-year training programme in an approved hospital training school, followed by written, practical and oral examinations. In theory the GNC was given the power to withdraw approval from inadequate training schools, but in practice hospitals simply appealed to the Ministry of Health to have these decisions overturned. The need to staff hospitals relegated training to a secondary concern, and the GNC endorsed policies that were economically driven rather than professionally motivated.

For nursing sisters and VADs who had earned their spurs in the mud of the Somme, such political wrangling seemed trite – futile and meaningless. In all probability, VADs who had worked at St John's were far more experienced than trained nursing sisters serving in civilian hospitals. Yet their unique and valuable experience in war counted for nothing in the civilian nursing field. They were still expected to complete a three-year training course in order to become registered. A few were consoled, however, by the earlier recognition afforded to them by the Order of St John. They had been made honorary nursing sisters of the Order, and that was all the status they needed.

Lily married Andrew in April 1919. Andrew continued his military career, and Lily bore four sons. Cynthia and Daisy undertook nurse training. Emma became an artist. Veronica lived in Paris directly after the war and had an eventful career in art and drama. Sisters Bemrose, Warner and McGinnis returned to civilian nursing and kept in touch with each other. Matron and Chitty remained close friends and also returned to civilian nursing. Many of these nurses did not marry. This was not unusual. Thousands of women became elderly spinsters during the interwar years because Britain had lost a whole generation of men. In total British war dead amounted to 888,246. To date, the Battle of the Somme remains one of the most enormous and gory conflicts in the history of war.

Appendix: Medal Citations

Military Medals

Matron Constance Elizabeth Todd, RRC, St John's Ambulance Brigade Hospital
For gallantry and devotion to duty during an enemy air raid. She moved freely about the wards during the bombing encouraging sisters and patients, and displayed great bravery and presence of mind throughout.

Assistant Matron Mabel Chittock, St John's Ambulance Brigade Hospital
For gallantry and devotion to duty during an enemy air raid. She displayed great presence of mind and instilled courage and confidence throughout a very trying time.

Sister Catherine Warner, St John's Ambulance Brigade Hospital
For gallantry and devotion to duty during an enemy air raid. She displayed the utmost coolness and maintained a cheery spirit throughout showing great bravery.

Sister Jane Bemrose, St John's Ambulance Brigade Hospital
For gallantry and devotion to duty during an enemy air raid. She showed disregard for danger and continued to attend to the wounded in her charge during heavy bombardment.

Sister Molly McGinnis, St John's Ambulance Brigade Hospital
For gallantry and devotion to duty during an enemy air raid.
She showed great courage, took charge of a ward and sustained
her patients.

*Sister Margaret Hendebourck Ballance, St John's Ambulance
Brigade Hospital*
For gallantry and devotion to duty during an enemy air raid.
Her fortitude and courage were most conspicuous. She devoted
herself entirely to her patients.

Mentioned in dispatches for acts of bravery:
Sister A.W. Bain 30–12–18, posthumous
Sister M.A. Batey 4–1–17
Matron C.E. Todd 15–6–16
Miss D.J. Gould 29–5–17
Miss H. Trimble 29–5–17
Sister A.H. Murray 1–11–17
Sister N.S. Worsley 30–12–18
Miss E. Patchett 30–12–18
Miss E.M. White 30–12–18
Colonel C.J. Trimble 5–6–16, 21–12–17, 30–12–18 and 10–7–19
Captain F. Hall 30–12–18
Captain W. Wilson 30–12–18
Major C.M. Hope 30–11–18 and 10–7–19
Major T. Houston 1–11–17, 30–11–18 and 10–7–19

Life Saving Medals of the Order Of St John

GOLD: Colonel C.J. Trimble, CB, CMG, RAMC
During the severe air raids that occurred on the 19 and
31 May 1918 Colonel Trimble was constantly passing through
the various departments and entrenchments of the hospital,
encouraging the patients and personnel and directing

operations. It was largely due to the fact that he displayed such coolness and disregard for his own personal safety that so many escaped injury and no panic occurred. On one occasion he was knocked over and slightly wounded by a bomb which burst 3 feet from where he was standing. On another occasion a fire broke out after the bursting of a bomb and this was extinguished by the personal assistance of Colonel Trimble.

SILVER: Captain Frederick Hall, RAMC
Captain Hall was on duty in his ward when the St John Ambulance Brigade Hospital at Étaples was bombed on the 31 May 1918. His great bravery and devotion to duty were very evident during the most terrible experience. He worked continually amongst the patients until his ward was ultimately blown up and he himself was severely injured by the debris. This officer displayed the greatest coolness and self-sacrifice during what was really a terrible time and his action and bearing is worthy of all praise.

SILVER: Captain William Wilson R.A.M.C.
Captain Wilson displayed great courage and determination working amongst the patients until his ward was absolutely blown to pieces by a large bomb. His bravery was a fine example of what a brave man can do. Though injured himself, he extricated two sisters and attended to them, carrying one who was suffering from a fracture of a leg, a distance of some 200 yards to the trenches in which the sisters and VADs were sheltering. On arrival there, and after putting the sisters in a safe place, he fainted.

N.B. Medal citations recorded in archives of St John also correlated with National Archive medal role – N.A. PRO/ WO329/2316

INDEX

If you enjoyed this book, you may also be interested in …

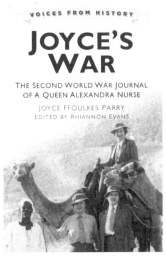
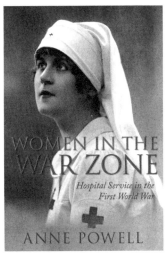